EVALUATION ETHICS
FOR BEST PRACTICE

EVALUATION ETHICS
FOR BEST PRACTICE

CASES AND COMMENTARIES

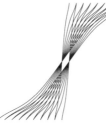

edited by

Michael Morris

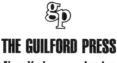

THE GUILFORD PRESS
New York   London

© 2008 The Guilford Press
A Division of Guilford Publications, Inc.
72 Spring Street, New York, NY 10012
www.guilford.com

Printed in the United States of America

This book is printed on acid-free paper.

Last digit is print number: 9   8   7   6   5   4   3   2   1

Library of Congress Cataloging-in-Publication Data

Evaluation ethics for best practice : cases and commentaries / edited by
Michael Morris.
    p. cm.
  Includes bibliographical references and index.
  ISBN-13: 978-1-59385-569-7 (pbk.: alk. paper)
  ISBN-10: 1-59385-569-9 (pbk.: alk. paper)
  ISBN-13: 978-1-59385-570-3 (hardcover : alk. paper)
  ISBN-10: 1-59385-570-2 (hardcover : alk. paper)
    1. Evaluation research (Social action programs)—Moral and ethical
aspects. I. Morris, Michael, 1949–
  H62.E8472 2008
  177—dc22
                                                            2007027511

Preface

What would you do if you encountered an ethical problem in your work as a program evaluator? One hopes, of course, for wisdom as well as for the courage that may be needed in order to "do the right thing." In practice, however, the challenge of doing the right thing does not present itself in the abstract but rather in the concrete circumstances of specific evaluations. This book focuses on concrete circumstances. A dozen case scenarios, half of which are accompanied by commentaries authored by pairs of respected evaluators, serve as the vehicle for ethical analysis. The chapters devoted to the scenarios represent each of the major stages of an evaluation, from the entry/contracting phase to utilization of results.

Our commentators were given a uniform set of questions to guide their examination of the cases. The key questions were:

- What are the major ethical issues raised by the case, when viewed from the vantage point of the Guiding Principles for Evaluators?
- Are there ethical dimensions to the case that are *not* covered by the Guiding Principles for Evaluators?
- If you were the evaluator in this case, what would you do, and why would you do it?
- What lessons, ethical and otherwise, might be drawn from the case?

Within this framework, commentators were free to develop their analyses as they saw fit. Some chose to add details to the scenario to provide a firmer grounding for their exploration of the case. Others employed their gift for novelistic narration or humorous metaphor when fashioning their presentation. The result, I am pleased to report, is a very thought-provoking set of essays on evaluation ethics.

When reading the commentaries, it is important to keep in mind that each one was prepared independently. For example, neither commentator on The Coordination Project scenario knew what the other was writing. This approach maximizes the diversity of the perspectives offered and adds to the richness of the commentaries as a group. As you will see, sometimes our contributors agree and sometimes they do not.

To make the initial scenario in each chapter more valuable for analysis and discussion, a "What if . . . ?" box accompanies those cases. Each box modifies the details of the scenario in three different ways. The question for readers to consider is whether, and how, these alterations change the ethical landscape of the case for the evaluator in terms of the issues to be addressed and the evaluator's response to those issues. (Note: The "What if . . . ?" boxes were not presented to commentators.) In other words, what are the differences that make an ethical difference, and what are the ones that don't? Understanding such distinctions is an important skill for evaluation practice.

The second case in each chapter—the one without commentaries—is followed by a set of questions designed to focus attention on key ethical issues raised by the scenario.

Good evaluators know how to ask good questions, and the same principle applies to case analysis. Keeping the following questions in mind when reviewing the scenarios will maximize the learning that can be extracted from them:

- What do I know for sure about this case?
- What, if anything, can I safely assume is true about the case?
- How do the circumstances of the case engage me in ethical terms both professionally and personally? How do my background and experience influence my reactions to the scenario?
- Do I need additional information about the case before I can make a substantive ethical decision? If so, how would I go about gathering that information?
- What obstacles am I likely to encounter when attempting to implement my decision? How can I deal with them?

These questions, of course, are useful not just for analyzing hypothetical scenarios but also for organizing one's thinking about the real-life ethical dilemmas that are faced when conducting evaluations. To the extent that the cases and commentaries in this book assist evaluators in developing the understanding, skill, and confidence necessary for ethical practice, they will have served their purpose.

ACKNOWLEDGMENTS

Without the insightful and stimulating contributions from our 13 commentators, this volume would not exist. Indeed, it is the high quality of these essays that makes me so proud to be associated with this book. In addition, the scenarios that appear *without* commentaries represent, in some cases, adaptations of ideas suggested by the commentators, specifically Michael Hendricks, Laura Leviton, Karen Kirkhart, Mel Mark, and Mary Ann Scheirer. I offer a special thank-you to those colleagues.

This book has benefited substantially from the thoughtful reviews provided by the following: William Bickel (University of Pittsburgh), Geni Cowan (California State University, Sacramento), Mark Hawkes (Dakota State University), Beth Menees Rienzi (California State University, Bakersfield), Hallie Preskill (Claremont Graduate University), John Schuh (Iowa State University), and Don Yarbrough (University of Iowa). Many of their suggestions were incorporated into this volume, and I am very grateful for them.

The genesis of this book resides in an invitation I received from C. Deborah Laughton at The Guilford Press. Simply put, C. Deborah Laughton is an author's dream come true. Supportive, wise, responsive, witty, and a consummate professional in the fine art of publishing, she makes the journey from prospectus to "in print" so painless that it's almost magical. Thank you, C. Deborah.

Contents

CHAPTER ONE

Ethics and Evaluation

"What you have done is highly unethical!"

These are words that no one likes to hear. They are especially troubling to individuals who see themselves as "professionals." Professionals are supposed to uphold the *highest* standards of behavior in their work. Accusations of unethical conduct suggest that exactly the opposite is occurring. Moreover, when framed in terms of individual behavior, discussions of ethical and unethical conduct are closely linked to judgments of moral accountability and character. Words like "should," "ought," and "must" enter into the conversation. Thus, it is not surprising that discussions of ethics have the ability to make us nervous, defensive, and annoyingly self-righteous. Moral accountability is a high-stakes affair.

This book focuses on ethical challenges in the emerging profession of program evaluation. Although definitions of evaluation abound in the literature, the one offered by Rossi, Lipsey, and Freeman (2004) is particularly well suited to our purposes: "**Program evaluation** is the use of social research methods to systematically investigate the effectiveness of social intervention programs in ways that are adapted to their political and organizational environments and are designed to inform social action to improve social conditions" (p. 16). This definition places evaluation within a broad context of reciprocal influence and utilization, implicitly highlighting the myriad opportunities for ethical difficulties to arise.

1

The core of the volume consists of a series of case study scenarios that end at a point at which the evaluator faces a decision about how to proceed, a decision that can be seen as having significant ethical ramifications. Each case is independently analyzed by two distinguished evaluators who offer insights concerning what the evaluator might do and why, using the American Evaluation Association's (AEA's) Guiding Principles for Evaluators as a framework for organizing their commentary. An equal number of case scenarios are presented without commentaries, so that readers can gain experience in developing ethical analyses without the "experts" looking over their shoulders. To provide a framework for our consideration of all the scenarios, we first explore, at a general level, how the domain of ethics intersects with program evaluation.

WHAT IS AN ETHICAL ISSUE?

A glance at the dictionary indicates that ethics deal with "what is good and bad and with moral duty and obligation" (*Webster's Ninth New Collegiate Dictionary*, 1988, p. 426). Newman and Brown (1996, p. 20) point out that three interrelated meanings are usually associated with the term *ethics*. The first focuses on fundamental principles of moral behavior that should apply, at least in theory, to everyone. The second refers to principles of conduct developed by, and for, members of a particular profession. The third involves the *systematic study* of the beliefs people hold, and the behaviors they exhibit, relevant to morality. All three meanings are relevant to our examination of ethical challenges encountered by evaluators. Professional codes for evaluators, such as the Guiding Principles for Evaluators, are specific applications of more basic ethical principles, and research on evaluation ethics (e.g., on ethical conflicts encountered by evaluators) can enhance our understanding of the arenas where ethical guidance is most urgently needed.

Given these definitions of ethics, it might appear that the distinction between what is and what is not an ethical issue should be pretty clear-cut. That is, ethical problems deal with matters of *moral* accountability related to "doing the right (good) thing" or "doing the wrong (bad) thing," while nonethical problems are ones where this dimension is not relevant. However, in practice, the line between ethical and nonethical concerns can frequently blur. What one evaluator views as an ethical issue might be perceived as simply a political problem, a philosophical disagreement, or a methodological concern by another. For example, in a study by Morris and Jacobs (2000), a national sample of evaluators read a case vignette in which a researcher only provided for minimal involvement of a community-based advisory board in an evaluation of an urban crime prevention program. Of the 49% of the sample that believed the researcher's behavior was *not* ethically problematic, half (50%) did not even think the vignette raised an ethical issue. Rather, they saw the scenario as posing methodological or philosophical concerns. In contrast, among the 39% of the sample that did regard the researcher's actions as ethically troublesome, one of the most frequent reasons given for this conclusion was that meaningful stakeholder participation represented a given in an ethical evaluation.

Disagreements about whether a particular problem does, or does not, represent an ethical conflict are not confined to evaluators (e.g., O'Neill & Hern, 1991). Unfortunately, our understanding of the factors that influence one's tendency to view professional problems through an ethical lens is not well developed. All we can say with certainty at this point is that significant individual differences exist.[1] Some might characterize these differences as variation in "moral sensitivity," which is "the ability to recognize the ethical dimensions of a situation" (Welfel & Kitchener, 1992, p. 179). Framing the issue in terms of ability, however, suggests that the key dimension involved is analytical competence, when it may be the case that factors such as value orientations and ideology play a much more prominent role.

It is against this background that the high-stakes consequences of defining problems in ethical terms are worth revisiting. By their very nature, ethical analyses of problems impose a moral burden on the actor ("What is the ethical thing for me to do in this situation?"). Analyses that are not couched in ethical terms impose no such burden (e.g., "Politically, what would be the most advantageous thing for me to do in this situation?"). The weight of a moral burden increases dramatically whenever the "ethical thing to do" could put the actor at risk, either personally or professionally. In these circumstances, there is much to be gained from *not* conceptualizing a problem as an ethical one. Implicitly if not explicitly, nonethical frameworks legitimize a much wider range of potential actions, including actions that do not put the decision maker at risk. How much of a role these motivational dynamics play in accounting for individual differences in viewing problems in ethical terms is not known. The more general point underscored by this discussion, however, is that the question "What is an ethical issue?" can be much easier to answer in theory than it often is in practice.

Ethical Dilemmas versus Mixed Dilemmas

Assuming that, in a given instance, we can agree that a particular problem does, in fact, constitute an ethical conflict, it is important to recognize the *type* of conflict it represents. MacKay and O'Neill (1992) distinguish between ethical dilemmas and mixed dilemmas. The former describes a situation in which there is a perceived conflict between two or more ethical principles, such as commitment to individual confidentiality versus responsibility for the overall public good. For example, an evaluator might discover evidence of serious wrongdoing while conducting confidential interviews. When faced with an ethical dilemma, one has to decide which ethical principle should be accorded higher priority when taking action.

In mixed dilemmas, *external factors* make it difficult or challenging to honor one or more ethical principles in practice. Consider the case of an evaluator being pressured by a stakeholder to write a report that portrays the accomplishments of the stakeholder's program more positively than is warranted by the data. The conflict here is between the principle of honesty/integrity and the political influence that the stakeholder is attempting to exert.

It is usually clear to the individual in a mixed dilemma what it is, from an ethical perspective, he or she *should* do. The problem is that the ethical course of action is often a risky course of action for that individual. The evaluator who refuses to bend in response to stakeholder pressure for positive results might find him- or herself the target of a subtle (or not so subtle) smear campaign waged by the aggrieved stakeholder ("Evaluator X is really difficult to work with"). In contrast, in pure ethical dilemmas, it is the lack of clarity about what should be done that is at the heart of the dilemma (although the challenge of how best to *implement* the particular "what" that is eventually chosen can, in many cases, remain). Should the evaluator honor the confidentiality of the source that informed the evaluator of the wrongdoing, or does the evaluator's responsibility to the greater good require that confidentiality be broken? Evaluators, therapists, and other professionals have debated such issues for decades (e.g., Cooksy, 2000; Huprich, Fuller, & Schneider, 2003; Knott, 2000; Morris, 2000; Sieber, 1994).

Determining what type of dilemma an ethical conflict represents is a valuable analytical skill, because figuring out *what* one is going to do is a different task than figuring out *how* one is going to do it. The former task is the primary concern of ethical dilemmas, whereas the latter is more closely associated with mixed dilemmas. Becoming proficient at both tasks is necessary for evaluators who wish to deal effectively with the ethical challenges they face.

ETHICAL PRINCIPLES

Having conceptualized ethical issues as an overall domain, the next step is to identify frameworks that strive to provide guidance to those who wish to behave ethically. Although the focus of this book is on ethical problems encountered by evaluators, it is critical to place these problems within the context of a discussion of ethical principles in general. In *Applied Ethics for Program Evaluation*, Newman and Brown (1996) examine five ethical principles identified by Kitchener (1984) as being relevant to the helping professions and suggest that these principles are applicable to evaluation as well.

Respect for Autonomy

Briefly stated, autonomy is the "right to act freely, make free choices, and think as you wish" (Newman & Brown, 1996, p. 38). In exercising this right, of course, we are obligated to respect the autonomy of others. An evaluator's desire to gather information, for example, does not necessarily override someone else's right *not* to provide some or all of that information, depending on the circumstances.

Nonmaleficence

This is probably the most widely known ethical principle subscribed to by professionals: "Do no harm." The goal here is to avoid inflicting physical or psychological injury on others and, whenever possible, to protect them from exposure to the *risk* of harm. In situations in which harm is likely or unavoidable, the principle of nonmaleficence requires us to take steps to minimize that harm and to have a reasonable expectation that the harm experienced will be more than compensated for by the benefits (direct and indirect) generated by our actions. Thus, an evaluator who gathers information on sensitive topics should attempt to minimize respondents' stress and discomfort and, depending on the issues being addressed, provide respondents with information about services that could be beneficial to them (e.g., Stiffman, Brown, Striley, Ostmann, & Chowa, 2005).

Beneficence

This principle holds that we have a responsibility to do good, to be helpful to others in a proactive sense. Although philosophers may disagree over whether beneficence represents a duty or a virtue (e.g., Frankena, 1973), it is certainly the case that professionals in many fields are expected to be beneficent in their interactions with clients and other stakeholders. Evaluators, for example, are expected to conduct research in a way that provides stakeholders with the "best possible information" (American Evaluation Association, 2004, Preface-B) to facilitate decision making about programs.

Justice

The principle of justice encompasses at least two dimensions. The first, procedural justice, concerns the fairness of *how* decisions are made that affect the lives of others. The second, distributive justice, focuses on fairness in the allocation of *outcomes* (e.g., benefits, punishments) to individuals and groups.

In general, one would expect procedural justice to result in distributive justice, but exceptions are clearly possible. For instance, a needs assessment might gather data from a stratified random sample of community residents for the purpose of program planning. Despite the best efforts of the researchers, however, recent changes in the community's demographic profile result in certain subgroups being underrepresented in the needs assessment's findings. Consequently, the programs (i.e., outcomes) generated by the study turn out not to be responsive to the distinctive needs of the undersampled subgroups. In this case, a good faith attempt to achieve procedural justice (i.e., use of a stratified sample) did not succeed in producing distributive justice.

Fidelity

To display fidelity is to be faithful, which, in practice, translates into "keeping promises, being loyal, and being honest" (Newman & Brown, 1996, p. 49). Describing someone as acting "in good faith" is one way of claiming that he or she is upholding the principle of fidelity. An evaluator who agrees to facilitate a series of feedback meetings for various stakeholder groups after submitting a final report, and then proceeds to do so despite encountering a crisis in his or her personal life during that period, is demonstrating a high level of fidelity. Fidelity and integrity are similar concepts in that both emphasize steadfastness and commitment. Fidelity in this context, however, tends to be used more often when the focus is on commitment to *people*, whereas it is adherence to a set of *values* (e.g., moral principles) that generally is central in the case of integrity.

Any given action can, of course, be simultaneously relevant to two or more of these five principles. Thus, the evaluator who follows through with the feedback sessions is showing not only fidelity but also beneficence (by helping stakeholders understand and work with the evaluation's findings) and justice (by ensuring that the benefits of understanding are distributed fairly among all the stakeholder groups). When an action upholds all of the principles to which it is relevant, its ethical legitimacy is self-evident. However, as our discussion of ethical dilemmas indicated, there can be occasions when a particular behavior is consistent with one principle but not another. Consider, for example, a situation in which there are strong reasons to believe that disadvantaged (e.g., low-income) participants will benefit much less from an intervention than advantaged ones (e.g., Ceci & Papierno, 2005). Although both stakeholder groups are likely to be helped by the intervention, thus ensuring beneficence, the distribution of benefits is likely to *increase* the gap between the advantaged and the disadvantaged. If participating in an evaluation of this intervention is just as burdensome for the disadvantaged as the advantaged (or perhaps even more burdensome), it might be argued that the evaluation violates the principle of justice: The disadvantaged derive fewer benefits from their participation in the study, especially compared with the costs they incur, than the advantaged.

PROFESSIONAL GUIDELINES FOR ETHICAL EVALUATION PRACTICE

As the field of evaluation has evolved over the past half-century, it has increasingly taken on the characteristics of a profession (e.g., Fitzpatrick, Sanders, & Worthen, 2004; Smith, 2003; Worthen, 2003). One such characteristic has been the establishment of standards and principles to provide guidance to evaluators as they carry out their work in a wide variety of settings (Stufflebeam, 2003). In addition to the United States, countries and regions where evaluation standards have been developed include Canada, France, Germany, Switzerland, United Kingdom, Africa, Australia, and New Zealand (Picciotto, 2005; Russon & Russon, 2004). The most prominent guidelines in the United

States are the Guiding Principles for Evaluators (American Evaluation Association, 1995, 2004) and the Program Evaluation Standards (Joint Committee on Standards for Educational Evaluation, 1994).

The Guiding Principles for Evaluators

The Guiding Principles for Evaluators are designed to be relevant to all types of evaluations. There are five principles, each consisting of a very general statement accompanied by a more detailed description elaborating on the meaning and application of the principle. (See Appendix A for the full text of the Guiding Principles.)

- **Systematic Inquiry:** Evaluators conduct systematic, data-based inquiries.
- **Competence:** Evaluators provide competent performance to stakeholders.
- **Integrity/Honesty:** Evaluators display honesty and integrity in their own behavior and attempt to ensure the honesty and integrity of the entire evaluation process.
- **Respect for People:** Evaluators respect the security, dignity, and self-worth of respondents, program participants, clients, and other evaluation stakeholders.
- **Responsibilities for General and Public Welfare:** Evaluators articulate and take into account the diversity of general and public interests and values that may be related to an evaluation.

These principles reflect, to varying degrees, issues raised by Kitchener's ethical principles. Close alignment exists between Integrity/Honesty and fidelity, between Respect for People and respect for autonomy, and between Responsibilities for General and Public Welfare and justice. Nonmaleficence and beneficence seem to be relevant to all five Guiding Principles. One can easily imagine considerable harm resulting from a serious violation of any of the AEA principles. Similarly, upholding each of them is likely to enhance the evaluation's beneficence if one assumes that, in the long run, stakeholders and society in general are well served by high-quality, responsive evaluations.[2]

The Guiding Principles are classic examples of broad, overarching statements designed to sensitize evaluators to critical domains relevant to their work. The Systematic Inquiry principle focuses on the methodological dimension of evaluation. At its core, evaluation is a research endeavor, and evaluators have a responsibility to design and conduct studies that are technically sound and that adequately address the evaluation questions driving the project.

High-quality evaluations are not likely to occur if evaluators lack the "education, abilities, skills, and experience appropriate to undertake the tasks proposed in the evaluation" (American Evaluation Association, 2004, Principle B-1), which is the subject of the Competence principle. Because stakeholders frequently do not have the background to judge an evaluator's expertise, it is especially important that evaluators conscientiously assess the relevance of their qualifications to a particular project and act accordingly.

Cultural competence is also explicitly addressed by the Competence principle. Specifically, such competence is reflected in "evaluators seeking awareness of their own culturally-based assumptions, their understandings of the worldviews of culturally-different participants and stakeholders in the evaluation, and the use of appropriate evaluation strategies and skills in working with culturally different groups" (American Evaluation Association, 2004, Principle B-2). The topic of cultural competence has received growing attention in recent years, as researchers have begun to take seriously the challenge of conducting valid evaluations in settings and with populations whose values and norms differ significantly from their own (e.g., Bamberger, 1999; Monshi & Zieglmayer, 2004; Thompson-Robinson, Hopson, & SenGupta, 2004; see also Paasche-Orlow, 2004; Ramsey & Latting, 2005). Indeed, it is noteworthy in this regard that the original 1995 version of the Guiding Principles did not even include a discussion of cultural competence.

Evaluators must also display competence in their understanding of and adherence to laws and regulations relevant to the evaluations they conduct (e.g., the Family Educational Rights and Privacy Act, the Health Insurance Portability and Accountability Act). The regulatory environment of evaluation is becoming increasingly complex and demanding, as policies designed to protect research participants continue to be developed and elaborated on and are interpreted by various oversight groups (e.g., institutional review boards).

The basic theme underlying the Guiding Principle of Integrity/ Honesty is transparency. Evaluators should strive to ensure that stakeholders have a full understanding of the key issues addressed and decisions reached throughout the evaluation, including a consideration of the study's limitations and weaknesses. Of special significance here are concerns surrounding conflicts of interest and the undistorted communication of evaluation procedures, findings, and interpretations. With respect to conflict of interest, the principle indicates that "evaluators should disclose any roles or relationships they have that might pose a conflict of interest (or appearance of a conflict) with their role as an evaluator. If they proceed with the evaluation, the conflict(s) should be clearly articulated in reports of the evaluation results" (American Evaluation Association, 2004, Principle C-2).

A conflict of interest exists "when the personal or financial interests of an evaluator might either influence an evaluation or be affected by the evaluation" (Joint Committee on Standards for Educational Evaluation, 1994, p. 115). As Friedman (1992) wisely points out, having a conflict of interest is not, in and of itself, improper. He notes that "a conflict of interest exists whether or not decisions are affected by the personal interest; a conflict of interest implies only the potential for bias and wrongdoing, not a certainty or likelihood" (p. 246). From an ethical perspective, it is how evaluators (and others) *respond* to a conflict of interest that is crucial.

Conflicts of interest abound in professional life, and evaluation is no exception. Issues such as personal friendships with key stakeholders, providing input to the design of a program one is evaluating, and having one's future work prospects influenced by a stakeholder's reaction to the substance or tone of a final evaluation report are just three conflicts that evaluators must be prepared to deal with.

The Integrity/Honesty principle also maintains that "evaluators should not misrepresent their procedures, data or findings [and] within reasonable limits, they should attempt to prevent or correct misuse of their work by others" (American Evaluation Association, 2004, Principle C-5). Research indicates that being pressured to misrepresent findings is one of the most frequent challenges encountered by evaluators (Morris & Cohn, 1993). To the extent that evaluators can develop strategies for preventing stakeholder attempts to exert such pressure, the ethical terrain they traverse in their work will become much less hazardous.

The need to address misuse by others "within reasonable limits" highlights the limitations inherent in general pronouncements such as the Guiding Principles. Views of what constitutes reasonable limits can obviously differ, resulting in disagreements over what it is that evaluators are ethically required to do to minimize misuse.

The Guiding Principle of Respect for People encompasses issues that have traditionally been addressed under the rubric of "ethical treatment of human subjects," reflecting the Kantian categorical imperative that individuals must be treated as ends in themselves and not simply as means. These include topics such as informed consent, privacy and confidentiality, risk–benefit analysis, methods for selecting and assigning study participants, the use of deception, and incentives for participation (Cooksy, 2005; Oakes, 2002; U.S. Department of Health & Human Services, 1993). Although a detailed consideration of these issues is beyond the scope of this book, it should be noted that the multiple stakeholders involved in evaluation can greatly complicate the ethical analysis that must be undertaken in specific situations. Consider, for example, a pilot program for disruptive students that is offered within the public schools by an external agency. Key stakeholders are likely to include, at a minimum, the students in the program (including any control groups), the teachers of those students, the students' parents/guardians, students who interact with the disruptive students, program staff, school staff who interact with the disruptive students (e.g., counselors, social workers), and school administrators. An in-depth evaluation of this intervention will place different types, and different levels, of burdens on the various stakeholder groups, with the anticipated benefits to be derived from participating in the evaluation also varying substantially. Conducting a single cost–benefit analysis of the evaluation is almost certainly not going to be sufficient in this instance (see Mark, Eyssell, & Campbell, 1999). Evaluators cannot afford to think of human subjects as simply those who are members of experimental and control groups.

The fifth Guiding Principle, Responsibilities for General and Public Welfare, is the most provocative one from an ethical perspective. It claims that "evaluators have obligations that encompass the public interest and good" and that "because the public interest and good are rarely the same as the interests of any particular group . . . evaluators will usually have to go beyond analysis of particular stakeholder interests and consider the welfare of society as a whole" (American Evaluation Association, 2004, Principle E-5). Concepts such as the "public interest and good" and the "welfare of society" are not further specified or defined in the Guiding Principles, leaving room for myriad interpretations, many of them potentially conflicting. This, in turn, can result in conflicting perceptions of what constitutes ethical and unethical behavior. When one considers the various ideological perspectives that can be brought to bear on the question "What makes for a good society?," it becomes clear that what one evaluator views as an ethical issue, might be seen as simply a reflection of a broader political agenda by another. It may prove to be quite difficult in practice to achieve the goal, as one philosopher put it, of "distinguish[ing] ethics (as that which is concerned with questions of right and wrong) from politics (where our fundamental concern is to contest and clarify the nature of the collective good and bad)" (Checkland, 1996, p. 343). Indeed, some conceptualizations of evaluation explicitly link these two dimensions. Schwandt (2002), for example, regards evaluation as "first and foremost a . . . moral–political and interpretive practice, not a technical endeavor" (p. 196; see also Schwandt, 2007; Simons, 2006, pp. 255–256).

Along these lines, some theorists have explicitly grounded their notions of how evaluations should be conceptualized and conducted in a particular view of social justice. Deliberative democratic evaluation, advocated by House and Howe (1999, 2000), and empowerment evaluation (Fetterman & Wandersman, 2005) are two prominent examples. Other theorists, such as Schwandt (2007), stress the fundamental responsibility that evaluators have for *critically* examining the values, norms, and moral principles embodied in the programs they study. In other words, evaluators have an ethical responsibility to serve as proactive moral critics.

In a related vein, Blustein (2005) has asked, "When evaluating programs under federal support and with federal direction, is it acceptable to perform evaluations just as long as they are consistent with statutes, regulations, and congressional mandates? Are ethical questions put to rest by examining the legal issues?" (p. 840). These are crucial matters from a social justice perspective because the very act of evaluating a program can be seen by some as conferring a degree of legitimacy on the policy ideology underlying that intervention (e.g., Brodkin & Kaufman, 2000).

To be sure, the widespread adoption of social justice perspectives within the field would greatly expand the range of issues regarded as ethical in nature by evaluators. The more general point to be made here, however, is that the Guiding Principle of Responsibilities for General and Public Welfare erects a very large tent under which many different, and perhaps irreconcilable, ethical "verdicts" might be rendered, depending on the worldviews held by those applying the principle. Whatever that worldview may be, however, this principle suggests that evaluators should be mindful that their ethical responsibilities extend beyond the boundaries defined by their study's immediate stakeholders. Sorting out these responsibilities can be an exceedingly complex task and highlights the importance of being able to articulate clearly, to oneself and to others, the fundamental beliefs and values that guide one's work.

The Program Evaluation Standards

The Program Evaluation Standards (see Appendix B) "are intended to guide the design, employment, and critique of educational programs, projects, and materials" (Joint Committee on Standards for Educational Evaluation, 1994, p. 4). Although the reference here is to educational programs, the standards themselves are worded in a way that does not restrict their applicability to this particular domain. Indeed, the term *education* is not mentioned in *any* of the 30 Program Evaluation Standards (second edition, currently being revised). Thus, it is not surprising that the Program Evaluation Standards are frequently referenced in discussions of program evaluation ethics, both within and outside of education, and that many evaluators find the specificity of the standards (compared with the more general Guiding Principles for Evaluators) makes them particularly useful for analysis.

The second edition of the Program Evaluation Standards organizes them into four clusters, each reflecting an important attribute of an evaluation:

- **Utility:** These seven standards "ensure that an evaluation will serve the information needs of intended users" (Joint Committee on Standards for Educational Evaluation, 1994, p. 23).
- **Feasibility:** These three standards "ensure that an evaluation will be realistic, prudent, diplomatic, and frugal" (Joint Committee on Standards for Educational Evaluation, 1994, p. 63).
- **Propriety:** These eight standards "ensure that an evaluation will be conducted legally, ethically, and with due regard for the welfare of those involved in the evaluation, as well as those affected by its results" (Joint Committee on Standards for Educational Evaluation, 1994, p. 81).
- **Accuracy:** These 12 standards "ensure that an evaluation will reveal and convey technically adequate information about the features that determine worth or merit of the program being evaluated" (Joint Committee on Standards for Educational Evaluation, 1994, p. 125).

It is noteworthy that the word *ethical* only appears in the definition of the Propriety Standards, which deal with such matters as the rights of human subjects, protection from harm, informed consent, confidentiality, anonymity, conflicts of interest, disclosure of findings, and adherence to formal agreements (see Appendix B). However, given the research reviewed in subsequent sections of this chapter, one can make a compelling case that the standards in all four categories should be viewed as constituting a foundation for the ethical practice of evaluation.

Limitations of Professional Guidelines

Newcomers to evaluation, upon perusing the Guiding Principles for Evaluators and the Program Evaluation Standards, might conclude that they now have at their disposal an easy-to-follow road map for handling whatever ethical problems might come their way. Unfortunately, situations in which professional guidelines provide ready-made answers are likely to be the exception rather than the rule. Principles and standards are inherently general and abstract and thus cannot be fully responsive to the complexity and nuance encountered in specific circumstances. As Mabry (1999) has observed, "Codes of professional practice cannot anticipate the myriad particularities of ordinary endeavors. . . . Of necessity, practitioners must interpret and adapt them in application" (p. 199).

This process of adaptation often requires one to confront the challenge of favoring one professional principle or standard over another. The Guiding Principles, for example, are not prioritized. The authors of the Guiding Principles note that "priority will vary by situation and evaluator role [and that] sometimes these principles will conflict, so that evaluators will have to choose among them. At such times, evaluators must use their own values and knowledge of the setting to determine the appropriate response" (American Evaluation Association, 2004, Preface-E and Background). A major implication of this fact is that there are likely to be many cases in which an obsessive search for the one right answer to an ethical challenge in evaluation is ill-advised. There may be a number of right answers, each one representing a different combination of ethical pros and cons.

It is also important to remember that even when individuals perceive professional guidelines as providing unambiguous ethical advice, there is no guarantee that this advice will be followed. In clinical psychology, for example, Betan and Stanton (1999) note that "research repeatedly indicates a discrepancy between what psychologists define as the appropriate ethical decision [as defined by the American Psychological Association's ethics code] and their intention to implement the decision toward ethical action" (p. 295). Demographic factors do not play a significant role in explaining why some clinicians (and clinicians-in-training) are more likely than others to say that they *would* do what their professional code of ethics says they *should* do. In these situations, it appears that respondents often feel that their personal value systems should carry more weight in decision making than professional codes (e.g., Smith, McGuire, Abbott, & Blau, 1991). In other words, there is a willingness on the part of professionals to substitute their own value-based judgments for those rendered by professional codes, especially in cases in which personal values are seen as more contextually sensitive. Of course, there is also the possibility, noted earlier, that professional guidelines will not be adhered to because of the perceived risks associated with doing so.

What conclusions should evaluators draw from our analysis of professional guidelines? Probably the most significant one is that we should not expect more from the Guiding Principles for Evaluators or the Program Evaluation Standards than they are designed to deliver. As a "general orienting device" (Morris, 2003, p. 321), they can alert evaluators to the ethical issues they need to be mindful of, but specific strategies for resolving ethical dilemmas and mixed dilemmas are most likely to emerge from a detailed examination of the case at hand.

EVALUATORS' EXPERIENCES WITH ETHICAL CHALLENGES

When evaluators are asked about the ethical problems they have encountered in their work, what do they report? In the most comprehensive investigation of this issue, Morris and Cohn (1993) surveyed a random sample of the AEA membership, receiving responses from more than 450 individuals. Of this group, nearly two thirds (65%) indicated that they had faced ethical challenges when conducting evaluations; the remainder (35%) said they had not. Not surprisingly, the more experience one had in evaluation in terms of the number of evaluations conducted, the more likely it was that ethical conflicts were reported as having been encountered. External evaluators were also more likely than internal evaluators to say that they had faced ethical challenges in their work.

It is probably safe to assume that, within the group that reported no ethical problems, a certain percentage had encountered situations that other evaluators would have perceived as ethically troublesome. As we have seen, differences can exist among individuals in how they categorize the challenges they experience. In discussing their research on evaluation ethics, for example, Newman and Brown (1996) report that "we consistently found people whose generalized response was 'What? Ethics? What does ethics have to do with evaluation?' This came from experienced evaluators, long-time users of evaluation, evaluation interns, and faculty members teaching program evaluation" (p. 89). Given this background, perhaps it should not be shocking that more than one third of the Morris and Cohn sample claimed to have never grappled with an ethical problem in their evaluation work (see also Honea, 1992). Interestingly, in a survey of members of the Australasian Evaluation Society (Turner, 2003), 29% of the respondents indicated that they had never experienced an ethical problem in evaluation.

What Ethical Challenges Are Encountered?

At every stage of an evaluation, there are numerous opportunities for ethical problems to emerge. Analysis of the results of the Morris and Cohn study suggests that, in practice, some stages are more ethically hazardous than others. That is, when respondents were asked to describe the ethical challenges they encountered most frequently, the problems they reported tended to cluster in certain phases of the evaluation. An overview of these results follows.

Entry/Contracting Stage

This is the stage at which the evaluator and primary stakeholders engage in preliminary discussions of such issues as the need for, the nature of, and the feasibility of the proposed evaluation. During this phase, one of the key questions being considered by the evaluator is, "Should I take on this project?" Morris and Cohn's respondents identified a number of ethical problems associated with this stage:

- A stakeholder has already decided what the findings "should be" or plans to use the findings in an ethically questionable fashion.
- A conflict of interest exists.
- The type of evaluation to be conducted is not adequately specified or justified.
- A stakeholder declares certain research questions "off limits" in the evaluation despite their substantive relevance.
- Legitimate stakeholders are omitted from the planning process.

- Various stakeholders have conflicting expectations, purposes, or desires for the evaluation.
- The evaluator has difficulty identifying key stakeholders.

The first problem listed is an intriguing one. Apparently, it is not uncommon for evaluators to feel that they are being presented with a "done deal" during the entry/contracting phase, when the implicit (or not so implicit) message communicated by a stakeholder is "give me results that confirm X . . . or else." In other cases, it is clear that the primary stakeholder intends to use the evaluation to support a decision that has already been made. The decision might be to lobby for additional program resources, to terminate a program, or to release a staff member, to cite just three possibilities.

The second challenge confirms that conflicts of interest represent more than just an issue of hypothetical interest to evaluators. Respondents report instances in which they have experienced such a conflict as well as occasions when the conflicted party has been a stakeholder. Indeed, conflicts of interest have probably increased in recent years. For example, Nee and Mojica (1999) suggest that funders are increasingly asking for external evaluators' help in designing complex community initiatives that those same evaluators are supposed to evaluate, generating obvious concerns about conflicts of interest.

The third challenge indicates that the entry/contracting phase sometimes ends without a clear, detailed focus for the evaluation having been articulated. This state of affairs can set the stage for a host of problems later in the evaluation.

Another type of ethical conflict arises if a stakeholder wants to leave something out of an evaluation that the evaluator strongly believes should be included. For example, a stakeholder might be averse to having the evaluation explore the logic model underlying the program, despite (or perhaps because of) the evaluator's concern that the model may be seriously flawed.

The remaining entry/contracting problems all reflect the multiple-stakeholder nature of most evaluations. Evaluators can experience difficulty in locating relevant stakeholders; in convincing one stakeholder to welcome another stakeholder's participation in the evaluation; and in resolving disputes among stakeholders regarding the overall direction of the proposed evaluation. Dealing with these issues can be extremely challenging as the evaluator works through the question "Which stakeholder(s) do I owe primary allegiance to in this project?" As the Guiding Principles state, "Evaluators necessarily have a special relationship with the client who funds or requests the evaluation. . . . However, that relationship can also place evaluators in difficult dilemmas when client interests conflict with other interests" (American Evaluation Association, 2004, Principle E-4). These other interests, of course, include those of other stakeholders, and the Morris and Cohn data suggest that such dilemmas are no stranger to evaluators.

Designing the Evaluation

In the design phase, the methodology of the evaluation is developed. This methodology, of course, is influenced not just by technical concerns but also by political, cultural, logistical, financial, and ethical ones (ERS Standards Committee, 1982). The failure to gain acceptance of the overall evaluation design from all relevant stakeholders is the major ethical problem that Morris and Cohn's respondents reported in this phase. For example, an evaluator might feel pressured by stakeholders to adopt a design that the evaluator believes is methodologically inadequate. In certain cases, conflicts such as these can be viewed as an extension of some of the stakeholder-related difficulties described in the entry/contracting stage. If relevant stakeholders are not meaningfully engaged in the beginning, the chances that they will readily offer their full cooperation later might be severely diminished. For evaluators for whom stakeholder involvement is a high priority, this clearly poses an ethical, not just a political, problem.

Data Collection

Although informal data gathering begins with the first conversation between an evaluator and a potential evaluation client, "official" data collection is typically a product of the evaluation's formal design. The ethical problems that respondents mentioned most frequently in this stage fell into two categories. In the first, the rights or dignity of those providing data was compromised in some fashion. Difficulties in ensuring that data-collection procedures would protect the anonymity or confidentiality of evaluation participants were often the problem here. For example, the growing use of computerized databases in local, state, and federal agencies has made information sharing much easier, while also making it more difficult to protect the privacy of the often vulnerable populations profiled in those databases (e.g., Marquart, 2005).

The second issue involved situations in which the evaluator, in the course of data collection, discovered information pertaining to behavior that was illegal, unethical, or dangerous, thus raising the question of what, if anything, the evaluator should do with this information. It is not always clear what legal requirements the evaluator is subject to in these circumstances (Sieber, 1994). Even when such requirements are unambiguous, evaluators may feel an allegiance to ethical principles (e.g., honoring confidentiality) that conflict with them.

Data Analysis and Interpretation

In the data-analysis phase, the evaluator endeavors to make sense of the information gathered during the study. The potential impact of one's personal opinions and values on how the data are analyzed and presented is the major ethical challenge that Morris and Cohn's respondents identified during this stage (see also DeVries, Anderson, & Martinson, 2006). Respondents frequently felt that they were at risk of letting their personal views impair their objectivity. Even if one is skeptical of the ability of any researcher to be truly "objective," there is still the ethical problem of evaluators failing to explicitly acknowledge the role that their values may be playing in a given instance. This latter problem does *not* seem to be the one that concerned Morris and Cohn's respondents, however. Rather, they saw themselves struggling with the task of not allowing personal agendas to "contaminate" their analysis and understanding of the data (e.g., not letting their admiration for the goals or staff of the program distort their view of the program's impact).

Communication of Results

According to the respondents, this is the stage at which an evaluator is most likely to encounter an ethical conflict. The key problem here is the experience of being pressured by a stakeholder to misrepresent the evaluation's results. Indeed, this challenge is, by a wide margin, the study's most frequently reported ethical conflict. It is worth noting that such pressure also appears to be the conflict most often cited by respondents in the Australasian study (Turner, 2003). This pressure usually comes from the evaluation's primary client (but occasionally from the evaluator's superior), who wants the program portrayed in a more positive light (occasionally more negative) than the evaluator believes is warranted by the data. Sometimes disagreement focuses primarily on what the findings *mean* rather than on how positive or negative they are.

The changes that the stakeholder can attempt to bring about can range from relatively minor ("Is it possible to rework this sentence so that it comes across as a bit less harsh?") to substantial ("Those results should not be included in the report."). In the former case, the pressure is perhaps most accurately seen as presenting the evaluator with an *ethical* dilemma; the challenge is to display honesty and integrity in a way that is responsive to a stakeholder's legitimate needs ("do no harm"). When the changes desired are more significant, we are in the domain of *mixed* dilemmas; the evaluator believes that he or she is being asked to lie. Complicating the situation is that disagreement can exist over where the boundary is between a minor change and a major one. Moreover, in many instances, it may be in the stake-holder's self-interest to persuade the evaluator to view the latter as the former.

The other ethical challenges that evaluators report in the communication-of-findings stage concern confidentiality. Being pressured by a stakeholder to violate confidentiality is one problem. For example, a stakeholder might ask the evaluator to identify the source of a specific piece of information or request data sets that could permit identification. A second type of problem occurs when the evaluator is not pressured to violate confidentiality but is nonetheless concerned that reporting certain findings could represent a violation. This danger is greatest when the number of individuals providing data for the evaluation is relatively small. In these circumstances, the use of even the most general demographic characteristics to present findings can supply clues to the identities of specific respondents.

Utilization of Results

There is general acknowledgment within the field that evaluators are responsible for planning, conducting, and following up on their work in a fashion that maximizes the chances of the evaluation's findings being used by decision makers. Indeed, included in the Program Evaluation Standards are seven standards specifically devoted to the utility of the evaluation. It is important to recognize, however, that the evaluator's ability to directly influence the course of events is probably weakest during the utilization phase. Respondents reported a variety of ethical challenges during this stage:

- A stakeholder suppresses or ignores findings.
- Disputes or uncertainties exist concerning ownership/distribution of the final report, raw data, etc.
- A stakeholder uses the findings to punish another stakeholder or the evaluator.
- A stakeholder deliberately modifies findings before releasing them.
- A stakeholder misinterprets the findings.
- A stakeholder engages in plagiarism/misrepresentation of authorship (the accused party is usually the respondent's supervisor).

It is noteworthy that the most frequently cited problem is nonuse of findings. This is vivid testimony that, in the eyes of many evaluators, utilization represents an ethical issue for the evaluator and not just the stakeholder. Of course, the potential for problems does not end once use occurs. Stakeholders might employ the results to penalize others (e.g., by terminating employment), or they might misrepresent, knowingly or inadvertently, the findings. Benign misunderstanding probably represents the easiest of these challenges for the evaluator to address. Dealing with the others is likely to be much more difficult, requiring some degree of risk taking and confrontation on the evaluator's part.

The challenges involving ownership/distribution and authorship concern issues that, at least in theory, are typically negotiated during the entry/contracting phase. To be sure, such negotiation does not guarantee that all parties will act in good faith throughout the evaluation or that misunderstandings will not develop later. However, the appearance of these two challenges in the utilization phase reinforces a crucial truth: Ethical problems that manifest themselves in an evaluation's later stages are often rooted in the failure to address key issues in the earlier ones.

Implications

The challenges voiced by Morris and Cohn's national sample represent, of course, just a subset of all the ethical conflicts that evaluators might encounter (cf. Turner, 2003). The significance of these particular challenges is that they are the ones evaluators say they encounter most frequently. The study thus identifies the places where ethical land mines are most likely to await the typical evaluator. The more knowledge that evaluators have of this hazardous terrain, the more safely they can traverse it. However, ethical challenges perceived by evaluators might differ significantly from those articulated by other participants in the evaluation process (Newman & Brown, 1996). Research on attribution theory indicates that individuals tend to externalize problems (i.e., to not view their own behavior as causing the difficulties they experience; Kelley, 1973). Thus, evaluators might be less likely than other stakeholders to identify ethical conflicts where it is the evaluator's actions that are problematic.

Viewed as a whole, it appears that the entry/contracting, communication-of-findings, and utilization-of-results stages are the ones where evaluators are most likely to see themselves facing ethical hazards. To what extent is it possible to prevent problems in the latter two stages by thorough discussion and planning in the earlier ones? We will explore this question in Chapter Eight.

EVALUATION APPROACHES AND ETHICS

A number of attempts have been made to categorize the various schools of thought that have developed about how evaluations should be conceptualized and conducted. Fitzpatrick et al. (2004), for example, identify five approaches: objectives oriented, management oriented, consumer oriented, expertise oriented, and participant oriented. Stufflebeam and Shinkfield (2007) examine 21 (!) different approaches, grouping them into four overall categories: questions and methods oriented, improvement/accountability oriented, social agenda/advocacy oriented, and eclectic. Christie (2003) has tackled the issue empirically, asking eight prominent evaluation theorists to generate statements capturing the essence of their orientations to evaluation practice on three dimensions: methods, values, and use. The theorists later completed a questionnaire based in part on these initial items, with the results indicating that two basic factors distinguished the theorists from one another: scope of stakeholder involvement and method proclivity. Christie's study seems to represent a solid foundation for considering how the model of evaluation one subscribes to might be linked to one's views of ethical issues in evaluation.

Scope of Stakeholder Involvement

At the high end of this continuum are evaluators who endorse the notion of "*stakeholders having a role in all aspects of an evaluation, from inception to conclusion"* (Christie, 2003, p. 18). In Christie's study, David Fetterman (e.g., Fetterman & Wandersman, 2005) anchored this end of the stakeholder involvement scale. Evaluators strongly committed to stakeholder involvement are probably more likely than their less committed colleagues to be ethically troubled by evaluations that do not solicit meaningful stakeholder input. Interestingly, none of the theorists in Christie's sample were opposed to stakeholder involvement. As Alkin (2003) notes, *"all* of the theorists evidenced substantial concern for stakeholder participation and . . . the differences between them were simply gradations of relative stakeholder participation. . . . Clearly, the notion of stakeholder involvement, at least in principle, is widely engrained in the formulations of evaluation theorists" (p. 82).

In contrast, Christie found that the practitioners in her study— evaluators of California's Healthy Start program—were much less uniform than the theorists in their commitment to stakeholder involvement. Thus, there is reason to suspect that extensive stakeholder participation may not be nearly as normative in the real world of evaluation practice as one would expect from reading the work of leading theorists. To the extent that this is the case, ethical concerns over the necessity for stakeholder engagement may resemble something of "an acquired taste" despite the existence of disciplinary principles and standards extolling its importance. Indeed, those who are low in commitment to extensive stakeholder engagement might actually regard such involvement as ethically *inappropriate*, claiming that it can threaten the objectivity of the evaluation.

Method Proclivity

The second dimension that emerged from Christie's investigation involves "the extent to which the evaluation is guided by a prescribed technical approach" (2003, p. 20). At the high end of this continuum are those who subscribe to a *"particular methodology that has as a feature predetermined research steps"* (p. 21), and at the low end are those who do not display such a commitment. Given the stringent methodological requirements associated with randomized experiments, it is not surprising that Robert Boruch (e.g., 1997) anchored the high end of the proclivity scale. Toward the midpoint were more qualitatively oriented theorists (e.g., Eisner, 2003). The scale's low end was anchored by Michael Patton, whose utilization-focused perspective is explicit in recommending a "problem-solving approach that calls for a creative adaptation to changed and changing conditions, as opposed to a technical approach, which attempts to mold and define conditions to fit preconceived models of how things should be done" (Patton, 1997, p. 131).

What might be the implications of method proclivity for ethical concerns? Insofar as one holds strong, deep-seated beliefs about proper methods for conducting evaluations, it raises the possibility that the failure to apply those techniques when they are seen as warranted will be viewed as ethically problematic. Evaluators with less of an intellectual (and perhaps emotional) investment in a particular approach might view such episodes as simply methodological or philosophical disputes rather than ethical ones. A similar point could be made about commitment to stakeholder involvement. The less salient this issue is for an evaluator, the more likely that it will be conceptualized in terms of methodological or philosophical *preferences* rather than as ethical *imperatives*.

It is also the case, of course, that the *purpose* of an evaluation can have ethical implications for stakeholder involvement and the methodology used in the study. Mark, Henry, and Julnes (2000), for example, delineate four specific purposes for evaluation: assessment of merit and worth; program and organizational improvement; oversight and compliance; and knowledge development. In order for an evaluation to generate credible information in a given domain, certain types of stakeholder involvement might be required (or might be inappropriate), and certain methodologies could be essential (e.g., consider the use of double-blind clinical trials in medicine). Thus, if an evaluation's purpose is program improvement, the failure to meaningfully engage program staff throughout the evaluation might be viewed as much more ethically suspect than if hypothesis testing and knowledge development were the overriding goals.

This discussion suggests that overall approaches to evaluation do have ethical significance, at least for those who vigorously identify with a particular model (or purpose) for evaluation. In Christie's study, however, only a minority (36%) of the Healthy Start evaluators "were within meaningful proximity of a theorist, indicating that most do not use frameworks aligned with a specific theoretical model" (2003, p. 33). The extent to which these results can be generalized to other groups of evaluation practitioners is unclear. Even so, these findings caution us not to assume that the ethical antennae of theorists and rank-and-file practitioners are tuned to exactly the same frequencies.

NOTES

1. For research on individual differences in perceptions of ethical problems in the business arena, see Reynolds (2006).
2. For a comparison of the Guiding Principles and Kitchener's principles that reaches different conclusions, see Newman and Brown (1996, p. 53).

REFERENCES

Alkin, M. C. (2003). Evaluation theory and practice: Insights and new directions. In C. A. Christie (Ed.), *The practice–theory relationship in evaluation* (New directions for evaluation, no. 97, pp. 81–89). San Francisco: Jossey-Bass.

American Evaluation Association. (2004). *Guiding principles for evaluators* (rev.). Available at *www.eval.org/Publications/GuidingPrinciples.asp*.

American Evaluation Association, Task Force on Guiding Principles for Evaluators. (1995). Guiding principles for evaluators. In W. R. Shadish, D. L. Newman, M. A. Scheirer, & C. Wye (Eds.), *Guiding principles for evaluators* (New directions for program evaluation, no. 66, pp. 19–26). San Francisco: Jossey-Bass.

Bamberger, M. (1999). Ethical issues in conducting evaluation in international settings. In J. L. Fitzpatrick & M. Morris (Eds.), *Current and emerging ethical challenges in evaluation* (New directions for evaluation, no. 82, pp. 89–97). San Francisco: Jossey-Bass.

Betan, E. J., & Stanton, A. L. (1999). Fostering ethical willingness: Integrating emotional and contextual awareness with rational analysis. *Professional Psychology: Research and Practice, 30*, 295–301.

Blustein, J. (2005). Toward a more public discussion of the ethics of federal social program evaluation. *Journal of Policy Analysis and Management, 24*, 824–846.

Boruch, R. F. (1997). *Randomized experiments for planning and evaluation: A practical guide.* Thousand Oaks, CA: Sage.

Brodkin, E. Z., & Kaufman, A. (2000). Policy experiments and poverty politics. *Social Service Review, 74*, 507–532.

Ceci, S. J., & Papierno, P. B. (2005). The rhetoric and the reality of gap closing: When "have-nots" gain but the "haves" gain even more. *American Psychologist, 60*, 149–160.

Checkland, D. (1996). Individualism, subjectivism, democracy, and "helping" professions. *Ethics and Behavior, 6*, 337–343.

Christie, C. A. (2003). What guides evaluation?: A study of how evaluation practice maps onto evaluation theory. In C. A. Christie (Ed.), *The practice–theory relationship in evaluation* (New directions for evaluation, no. 97, pp. 7–35). San Francisco: Jossey-Bass.

Cooksy, L. J. (2000). Commentary: Auditing the off-the-record case. *American Journal of Evaluation, 21,* 122–128.

Cooksy, L. J. (2005). The complexity of the IRB process: Some of the things you wanted to know about IRBs but were afraid to ask. *American Journal of Evaluation, 26,* 353–361.

DeVries, R., Anderson, M. S., & Martinson, B. C. (2006). Normal misbehavior: Scientists talk about the ethics of research. *Journal of Empirical Research on Human Research Ethics, 1,* 43–50.

Eisner, E. (2003). Educational connoisseurship and educational criticism: An arts-based approach to educational evaluation. In T. Kellaghan & D. L. Stufflebeam (Eds.), *International handbook of education evaluation: Part one. Perspectives* (pp. 153–166). Dordrecht, The Netherlands: Kluwer Academic Publishers.

ERS Standards Committee. (1982). Evaluation Research Society standards for program evaluation. In P. H. Rossi (Ed.), *Standards for evaluation practice* (New directions for program evaluation, no. 15, pp. 7–19). San Francisco: Jossey Bass.

Fetterman, D. M., & Wandersman, A. (Eds.). (2005). *Empowerment evaluation principles in practice.* Thousand Oaks, CA: Sage.

Fitzpatrick, J. L., Sanders, J. R., & Worthen, B. R. (2004). *Program evaluation: Alternative approaches and practical guidelines* (3rd ed.). Upper Saddle River, NJ: Pearson/Allyn & Bacon.

Frankena, W. K. (1973). *Ethics* (2nd ed.). Englewood Cliffs, NJ: Prentice-Hall.

Friedman, P. J. (1992). The troublesome semantics of conflict of interest. *Ethics and Behavior, 2,* 245–251.

Honea, G. E. (1992). *Ethics and public sector evaluators: Nine case studies.* Unpublished doctoral dissertation, University of Virginia.

House, E. R., & Howe, K. R. (1999). *Values in evaluation and social research.* Thousand Oaks, CA: Sage.

House, E. R., & Howe, K. R. (2000). Deliberative democratic evaluation. In K. E. Ryan & L. DeStefano (Eds.), *Evaluation as a democratic process: Promoting inclusion, dialogue, and deliberation* (New directions for evaluation, no. 85, pp. 3–12). San Francisco: Jossey-Bass.

Huprich, S. K., Fuller, K. M., & Schneider, R. B. (2003). Divergent ethical perspectives on the duty-to-warn principle with HIV patients. *Ethics and Behavior, 13,* 263–278.

Joint Committee on Standards for Educational Evaluation. (1994). *The program evaluation standards: How to assess evaluations of educational programs* (2nd ed.). Thousand Oaks, CA: Sage.

Kelley, H. H. (1973). The process of causal attribution. *American Psychologist, 28,* 107–128.

Kitchener, K. S. (1984). Intuition, critical evaluation and ethical principles: The foundation for ethical decisions in counseling psychology. *The Counseling Psychologist, 12*(3), 43–56.

Knott, T. D. (2000). Commentary: It's illegal and unethical. *American Journal of Evaluation, 21,* 129–130.

Mabry, L. (1999). Circumstantial ethics. *American Journal of Evaluation, 20,* 199–212.

MacKay, E., & O'Neill, P. (1992). What creates the dilemma in ethical dilemmas?: Examples from psychological practice. *Ethics and Behavior, 2,* 227–244.

Mark, M. M., Eyssell, K. M., & Campbell, B. (1999). The ethics of data collection and analysis. In J. L. Fitzpatrick & M. Morris (Eds.), *Current and emerging ethical challenges in evaluation* (New directions for evaluation, no. 82, pp. 47–55). San Francisco: Jossey-Bass.

Mark, M. M., Henry, G. T., & Julnes, G. (2000). *Evaluation: An integrated framework for understanding, guiding, and improving policies and programs.* San Francisco: Jossey-Bass.

Marquart, J. M. (2005, October). *Ethical issues in state-level evaluation settings.* Paper presented at the meeting of the American Evaluation Association, Toronto, Ontario, Canada.

Monshi, B., & Zieglmayer, V. (2004). The problem of privacy in transcultural research: Reflections on an ethnographic study in Sri Lanka. *Ethics and Behavior, 14,* 305–312.

Morris, M. (2000). The off-the-record case. *American Journal of Evaluation, 21,* 121.

Morris, M. (2003). Ethical considerations in evaluation. In T. Kellaghan & D. L. Stufflebeam (Eds.), *International handbook of educational evaluation: Part one. Perspectives* (pp. 303–328). Dordrecht, The Netherlands: Kluwer Academic.

Morris, M., & Cohn, R. (1993). Program evaluators and ethical challenges: A national survey. *Evaluation Review, 17,* 621–642.

Morris, M., & Jacobs, L. (2000). You got a problem with that? Exploring evaluators' disagreements about ethics. *Evaluation Review, 24,* 384–406.

Nee, D., & Mojica, M. I. (1999). Ethical challenges in evaluation with communities: A manager's perspective. In J. L. Fitzpatrick & M. Morris (Eds.), *Current and emerging ethical challenges in evaluation* (New directions for evaluation, no. 82, pp. 35–45). San Francisco: Jossey-Bass.

Newman, D. L., & Brown, R. D. (1996). *Applied ethics for program evaluation.* Thousand Oaks, CA: Sage.

Oakes, J. M. (2002). Risks and wrongs in social science research: An evaluator's guide to the IRB. *Evaluation Review, 26,* 443–479.

O'Neill, P., & Hern, R. (1991). A systems approach to ethical problems. *Ethics and Behavior, 1,* 129–143.

Paasche-Orlow, M. (2004). The ethics of cultural competence. *Academic Medicine, 29,* 347–350.

Patton, M. Q. (1997). *Utilization-focused evaluation: The new century text* (3rd ed.). Thousand Oaks, CA: Sage.

Picciotto, R. (2005, October). The value of evaluation standards: A comparative assessment. *Journal of MultiDisciplinary Evaluation, 3,* 30–59. Retrieved August 24, 2006, from *www.evaluation.wmich.edu/JMDE/.*

Ramsey, V. J., & Latting, J. K. (2005). A typology of intergroup competencies. *Journal of Applied Behavioral Science, 41,* 265–284.

Rossi, P. H., Lipsey, M. W., & Freeman, H. E. (2004). *Evaluation: A systematic approach* (7th ed.). Thousand Oaks, CA: Sage.

Russon, C., & Russon, G. (Eds.). (2004). *International perspectives on evaluation standards* (New directions for evaluation, no. 104). San Francisco: Jossey-Bass.

Schwandt, T. A. (2002). *Evaluation practice reconsidered.* New York: Peter Lang.

Schwandt, T. A. (2007). On the importance of revisiting the study of ethics in evaluation. In S. Kushner & N. Norris (Eds.), *Dilemmas of engagement: Evaluation development under new public management and the new politics* (pp. 117–127). New York: Elsevier.

Sieber, J. E. (1994). Issues presented by mandatory reporting requirements to researchers of child abuse and neglect. *Ethics and Behavior, 4,* 1–22.

Simons, H. (2006). Ethics in evaluation. In I. F. Shaw, J. C. Greene, & M. M. Mark (Eds.), *The SAGE handbook of evaluation* (pp. 243–265). Thousand Oaks, CA: Sage.

Smith, M. F. (2003). The future of the evaluation profession. In T. Kellaghan & D. L. Stufflebeam (Eds.), *International handbook of educational evaluation: Part one. Perspectives* (pp. 373–386). Dordrecht, The Netherlands: Kluwer Academic.

Smith, T. S., McGuire, J. M., Abbott, D. W., & Blau, B. I. (1991). Clinical ethical decision making: An investigation of the rationales used to justify doing less than one believes one should. *Professional Psychology: Research and Practice, 22,* 235–239.

Stiffman, A. R., Brown, E., Striley, C. W., Ostmann, E., & Chowa, G. (2005). Cultural and ethical issues concerning research on American Indian youth. *Ethics and Behavior, 15,* 1–14.

Stufflebeam, D. L. (2003). Professional standards and principles for evaluation. In T. Kellaghan & D. L. Stufflebeam (Eds.), *International handbook of educational evaluation: Part one. Perspectives* (pp. 279–302). Dordrecht, The Netherlands: Kluwer Academic.

Stufflebeam, D. L., & Shinkfield, A. J. (2007). *Evaluation theory, models, and applications.* San Francisco: Jossey-Bass.

Thompson-Robinson, M., Hopson, R., & SenGupta, S. (Eds.). (2004). *In search of cultural competence in evaluation: Toward principles and practices* (New directions for evaluation, no. 102). San Francisco: Jossey-Bass.

Turner, D. (2003). *Evaluation ethics and quality: Results of a survey of Australasian Evaluation Society members.* Retrieved September 2, 2006, from *www.aes.asn.au/about/ethics_survey_summary.pdf.*

U.S. Department of Health & Human Services. (1993). *IRB guidebook.* Retrieved September 1, 2006, from *www.hhs.gov/ohrp/irb/irb_guidebook.htm.*

Webster's ninth new collegiate dictionary. (1988). Springfield, MA: Merriam-Webster.

Welfel, E. R., & Kitchener, K. S. (1992). Introduction to the special section: Ethics education—an agenda for the '90s. *Professional Psychology: Research and Practice, 23,* 179–181.

Worthen, B. R. (2003). How can we call evaluation a profession if there are no qualifications for practice? In T. Kellaghan & D. L. Stufflebeam (Eds.), *International handbook of educational evaluation: Part one. Perspectives* (pp. 329–344). Dordrecht, The Netherlands: Kluwer Academic.

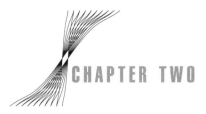

CHAPTER TWO

The Entry/Contracting Stage

The Coordination Project

As a researcher with experience in the evaluation of collaborative efforts between human service organizations, you have been contacted by the associate director of the state's Office of Child Protective Services (OCPS). Nearly 2½ years ago, OCPS initiated a project to improve coordination and case management among a number of agencies that provide services to neglected and abused youth. OCPS would like an evaluator to assess the extent to which the project has enhanced working relationships among the agencies involved. You are now meeting with the associate director to discuss the project in greater detail before submitting a formal evaluation proposal.

During the meeting, the associate director communicates her desire to have evaluation data collected from a wide variety of agency representatives, including staff from OCPS. You express agreement and also indicate your belief that the opinions and perspectives of service *consumers* (e.g., children, parents, guardians, foster families) could shed much-needed light on certain aspects of the success of the coordination project.

To put it mildly, the associate director does not share your view. In her opinion, the incorporation of consumer input into the study would dilute the

31

evaluation's focus and generate, in her words, "a laundry list of complaints and issues that are, at best, only marginally relevant to the purpose of this evaluation. They'll simply use the data gathering as an opportunity to vent about anything and everything, no matter how you structure the interview or survey. This just isn't the time or place for a study of client concerns. Your evaluation resources should be devoted to gathering as much in-depth information from staff as you can. They're the ones who've lived with this project most intimately over the past 2 years."

Although there are many responses you could offer to the associate director, the intensity with which she has expressed her objections makes you question your ability to fashion an argument that she would find persuasive. Indeed, at this point there is little doubt in your mind that inclusion of a "consumer component" in your evaluation proposal would seriously diminish the proposal's chances of being accepted by the associate director. On the other hand, you are convinced that any evaluation of the coordination project that does *not* include a consumer perspective will be seriously limited. Would this limitation be so damaging that it would undermine the fundamental validity and usefulness of the evaluation? If the evaluation sponsor wants a study that is narrower in scope rather than broader, isn't that her right?

As you ponder these questions, you ask yourself, "What is my responsibility as an evaluator in this situation?"

C O M M E N T A R Y

Consumers, Culture, and Validity

Karen E. Kirkhart

The evaluand (i.e., focus of the evaluation) in this scenario is a state-level OCPS project to improve "coordination and case management" of services for neglected and abused youth. The project has been ongoing for 2½ years, which places it solidly into implementation, making the evaluation request timely and appropriate. The associate director of OCPS, the identified client of the evaluation, wants to examine project impact on the working relationships among the agencies involved, presumably focusing on line workers, supervisors, and administrators. She wishes to exclude consideration of project impact on clients of case management services.

ETHICAL ISSUES

The major ethical concerns raised here involve validity. Construct underrepresentation—operationalization that is too narrow, omitting important dimensions—is a core source of invalidity (Messick, 1995). This case is fundamentally about construct underrepresentation (failures of omission) from two specific but related foci: the omission of consumer perspectives and the omission of culture. Casting validity as an ethical issue is not a new idea; ethics and validity have been understood as related for decades (Cronbach, 1988; Messick, 1980). This case illustrates well how ethical and methodological issues intertwine, a linkage made explicit in the Guiding Principle of Systematic Inquiry.

Omitting consumer perspectives creates ethical challenges in this scenario because of both the nature of the evaluation questions posed and the fundamental nature of the evaluand.

Nature of the Evaluation Questions

First, consider the questions that frame the proposed study. Such an approach is wholly consistent with the premises of the Systematic Inquiry principle, which directs evaluators to "explore with the client the shortcomings and strengths both of the various evaluation questions and the various approaches that might be used for answering those questions" (American Evaluation Association, 2004, Principle A-2).

The associate director frames the evaluation question in terms of the "working relationships among the agencies involved," narrowly operationalizing project outcomes in terms of enhanced interactions among staff and administration. Under this conceptualization, the focus of the evaluation is pure process, which includes immediate effects on staff members; that is, the impact that staff members have experienced during the operation of the coordination project itself. However, examining the logic behind service coordination reveals multiple constituencies impacted. The coordination project is designed to alter the behavior of staff members delivering services to neglected or abused youth and their caregivers within human service organizations. It affects service providers, who in turn affect consumers of services. The associate director is interested only in the impact on providers, arguing that the persons "who've lived with this project most intimately" are the staff of the participating agencies and programs. This is a questionable assumption; consumers have also had to live with the procedural changes, and nothing is more intimate than services that touch your family. Although it is certainly important to understand the intended impact of the project on providers' daily operations, it is also imperative to monitor its effects on those receiving OCPS services. Clearly, OCPS consumers—children, parents, guardians, foster families—are stakeholders in this evaluation; their systematic exclusion violates the principle of Responsibilities for General and Public Welfare, which calls for the inclusion of "relevant perspectives and interests of the full range of stakeholders" (American Evaluation Association, 2004, Principle E-1).

Questions about the success of the coordination project are inextricably linked to both provider behavior *and* impact on the consumer. The process of service coordination may abound with interesting and important issues, such as cost savings, time efficiency, or implications for privacy within information management, but the scenario poses a broader question when it asks, "Has case management improved?" This means that examining the coordination process alone is insufficient. Without consumer input, one cannot conduct a valid evaluation of whether case management has been enhanced. To put it bluntly, one cannot claim to understand improvement (or lack thereof) in case management by studying only half the picture—staff perceptions—while omitting the perspective of impacted recipients of service. Such a narrow representation of improvement would produce misleading conclusions, violating the Integrity/Honesty principle (American Evaluation Association, 2004, Principle C-6). The principle of Responsibilities for General and Public Welfare similarly cautions against narrowness in advising evaluators to "consider not only the immediate operations and outcomes of whatever is being evaluated, but also its broad assumptions, implications and potential side effects" (Principle E-2).

A sponsor opting for a study of narrow scope is not necessarily unethical; no single evaluation tackles all potentially relevant questions regarding a given evaluand. However, the nature of the evaluand must inform decisions regarding scope. The evaluator cannot systematically ignore information or omit a perspective that creates a partial, biased understanding and undermines validity. Given the nature of this particular evaluand, omitting consumers would have exactly that effect.

Nature of the Evaluand

Suppose the associate director simply narrowed her evaluation question further, omitting reference to improvement of case management. Would that erase the ethical challenge in this scenario? I would argue no because of the concern for public good that infuses child protective services and is reinforced by the principle of Responsibilities for General and Public Welfare. Because the context of this coordination project is the protection of vulnerable populations, omitting them from consideration in the evaluation is not an ethical option for two reasons. First, the evaluation should be congruent with the mission of OCPS as a human service organization, which is consumer protection. A limited construal of project impact closes off consideration of possible harm to consumers. Without the ability to examine harm as an unintended outcome of the coordination project, the evaluation falls short of its Responsibilities for General and Public Welfare.

Second, an evaluation that omits the consumer perspective may itself exert harm by reinforcing the powerlessness of the neglected and abused youth. This is a potent consequence that should not be minimized. These youth have experienced powerlessness in their home situations and again in the system that removed them from perceived danger. The evaluation should not replicate this neglect by failing to consider their experience as a case that was "managed" under the coordination project. The attitude expressed by the associate director intensifies this concern, because it communicates distance from and disrespect of the consumer, pointing to possible institutional discrimination. She expresses contempt for her clientele, portraying them as people with endless and presumably groundless complaints. This attitude is inconsistent with the principle of Respect for People, which directs evaluators to respect the "dignity and self-worth of . . . program participants [and] clients" (American Evaluation Association, 2004, Principle D).

Thus far, I have argued that excluding consumer perspectives poses a serious ethical issue and validity threat, but a second aspect of construct underrepresentation remains. Validity of evaluative conclusions is compromised by lack of attention to cultural context. These two concerns (consumer and cultural omissions) intersect, because the consumer population is arguably more diverse than the staff of OCPS. Omitting consumers, therefore, also limits the opportunity to represent cultural context accurately.

Fidelity to the component of the Competence principle involving cultural competence requires an understanding of cultural context. There are multiple layers of culture relevant to this case. Although the Competence principle approaches cultural diversity from the perspective of "culturally-different participants and stakeholders" (American Evaluation Association, 2004, Principle B-2), culture at the broader organizational or systems level is also relevant to evaluating the coordination project.

Organizational Culture

Organizational culture includes values, beliefs, history, and traditions that shape the local context of professional practice. Understanding these organizational variables is a prerequisite to valid inference and judgment concerning the coordination project. For example, what are the attitudes of staff members toward one another (both individually and collectively) and toward their consumer population? Do they share the associate director's contempt for consumers? Are there differences in attitude toward service recipients among the agencies being coordinated, and if so, whose values were elevated or suppressed in this project? What is the reward structure for recognizing meritorious performance among staff? How is power distributed among the agencies engaged in collaboration? Is there equity of workload and remuneration across member agencies? What is the history of stability versus restructuring among these agencies? Is there differential turnover in administration and staff across agencies? These and other markers of organizational culture set the context for understanding working relationships among the agencies involved.

Organizational culture is also shaped by context beyond the boundaries of the agencies. The Respect for People principle demands a comprehensive understanding of important contextual elements of the evaluation (American Evaluation Association, 2004, Principle D-1). In the coordination project, this includes legislative mandates and oversight, funding trends (expansion/reduction), mergers (or threats thereof), media coverage of incidents involving abused or neglected children, and the political context of OCPS services within the state. Elements of broader context that impact service delivery to consumers include changes in rules governing OCPS, demographic shifts in the population served, and increases/decreases in availability of placements or services.

Stakeholder Culture

The Respect for People principle is also explicit in addressing evaluators' responsibility to understand and respect differences among participants (American Evaluation Association, 2004, Principle D-6). This refers to evaluation participants as well as program participants. In this instance, it would refer to the personal characteristics of the workers and administrators implementing the coordination project as well as of the youth and their families or guardians and the foster families with whom they are placed.

The diversity dimensions of race, ethnicity, gender, religion, and social class addressed in the Competence principle (American Evaluation Association, 2004, Principle B-2) are relevant to both providers and consumers in this scenario. Children of all racial and ethnic backgrounds are subject to abuse and neglect but not at equal rates. The racial and ethnic distribution for the particular state in the scenario would need to be explored. For example, although national data suggest that one half of all child victims are White and one quarter are African American, an informal query of my local OCPS shows the proportion of Black and White families that are tracked is relatively equal. Race is also relevant among providers, with the majority of service providers (field staff and supervisors) being White. Boys and girls are abused at relatively equal rates, but within the OCPS workforce women sharply outnumber men. Most providers would be considered middle class, but their locations differ within this very broad category. Economic diversity among workers is reflected in the reward systems and hierarchies of salary and benefits within these service organizations as well as in workers' families of origin, which may range from poverty level to upper socioeconomic status. Among consumers, economic diversity is skewed, and families living in poverty are overrepresented.

Additional provider diversity lies in professional training and experience. What are their levels of education, disciplines in which they were trained, and years of experience in OCPS? Professional discipline relates to workers' obligations to honor various professional standards on culture (e.g., National Association of Social Workers, 2001). One cannot answer with confidence key evaluation questions concerning working relationships among providers without considering such cultural components. How has the collaboration project changed or left unchanged the faces of the workforce with whom both staff and consumers interact daily? Did it increase or decrease staff turnover? Did it deepen stereotypes or erase them? Expand or narrow workforce diversity?

On the consumer side, other important diversity variables "pertinent to the evaluation context" (American Evaluation Association, 2004, Principle B-2), singly and in interaction with one another, are family composition, sexual orientation, age, disability, education, and language spoken in the home. Family composition is a major consideration. Are caregivers in two-parent households treated with the same respect as single parents? Are same-sex parents being afforded the same respect and rights as heterosexual parents? How are extended families and nonbiological caregiver relationships treated? What are the economics of child protection: Who is supported and who is financially exploited? Age and physical or mental disability are relevant to both youth and their caregivers. What are the developmental and special needs of the children, and how well are these needs being met within the parameters of caregivers' age and abilities?

Culture reveals potential evaluation questions that are essential to valid inference and judgment concerning the coordination project. Does the coordinated system provide better access to appropriate translation, for example, or would a deaf family find it more difficult to communicate than under the prior model in which there was quite possibly greater worker specialization? If the new system is more efficient—defined as less time spent per family or more families served per time period—is this pace culturally congruent? The "inefficiencies" of the previous system may have permitted time for building relationships and trust, which have now been stripped from the coordinated model. Has the coordinated model increased or decreased the likelihood that a family of color will be working with someone who looks like them or who understands their circumstances? Will they have ready access to someone who is fluent in their primary language? If worker and client are not equally bilingual, whose language prevails?

Omission of culture strips full understanding, limiting the evaluator's ability to explore certain questions and clouding the answers to others by restricting the variables considered. Because the validity of inferences and evaluative judgments in multicultural contexts rests on multiple justifications, validity is also subject to multiple threats when culture is disregarded (Kirkhart, 1995, 2005). Neglecting culture constrains the theoretical foundations of the evaluation, the questions asked, the sources of evidence deemed legitimate, and the methods used to gather and analyze data. It undermines accurate synthesis and interpretation.

ETHICAL DIMENSIONS NOT ADEQUATELY ADDRESSED BY THE GUIDING PRINCIPLES

Although the Guiding Principles are intended to stimulate professional self-examination and discussion, there is not a specific principle that encourages evaluator self-reflection. The Integrity/Honesty principle directs evaluators to be explicit about their own "interests and values" (American Evaluation Association, 2004, Principle C-4), and the Competence principle notes that "cultural competence would be reflected in evaluators seeking awareness of their own culturally-based assumptions" (Principle B-2), but these issues merit greater attention and expansion. The Guiding Principles give insufficient attention to the need for evaluators to examine their own cultural position, agendas, and motivation.

Cultural characteristics that collectively map my personal location also position my work as an evaluator. I bring to this conversation my cultural identifications as a White, English-speaking, heterosexual, female academic. I am politically liberal and mature in years, a card-carrying member of both the American Civil Liberties Union and American Association of Retired Persons. I come from a working-class family of origin and was a first-generation college student. These and other dimensions that define me also position my potential evaluation of this program and my interaction with the associate director. They need to be recognized as they relate to this scenario in both direct and indirect ways. For example, my academic training is jointly in social work and psychology, which gives me guidance on both ethics and cultural competence from two professional vantage points. The Guiding Principles are explicit in respecting such discipline-based standards. I am a wife and mother; the latter is especially relevant to my values regarding the protection of children. My group memberships give me lenses through which I view my professional and personal life experiences, just as the persons with whom I interact have their individual frames of reference (Ridley, Mendoza, Kanitz, Angermeier, & Zenk, 1994).

The Coordination Project scenario raises the perennial question of whose agenda drives an evaluation. I notice my own reaction as evaluator to the associate director. I don't like this woman. Her manner strikes me as arrogant and inflexible. She wants to control the evaluation design, and she wants that design established concretely at the outset. I notice that this runs against my preference for emergent designs, in which elements can be added to follow leads that present themselves during the evaluation process. I also notice that, not only as an evaluator but as a social worker and community psychologist, I find her devaluing consumers offensive, and I wonder whether, consistent with her example, this attitude of disrespect permeates her workforce.

I must also scrutinize my own motivation with suspicion. Is my advocacy of consumer inclusion a knee-jerk, liberal reaction to the authoritarian style of the associate director? Am I getting drawn into a power struggle with her? Is my insistence on consumer inclusion itself well grounded in the best interests of the consumers? Or am I seeking to include them in ways that would place an additional burden on already overburdened family systems, potentially exploiting them to meet my own agenda? Consistent with the Respect for People principle, I see my overall position as respecting the dignity and self-worth of program clients; however, I have to be cognizant of the power differentials within this system and make sure that my advocacy of consumer inclusion is not, in fact, putting them at greater risk. Although the Respect for People principle addresses "risks, harms, and burdens that might befall those participating in the evaluation" (American Evaluation Association, 2004, Principle D-2), it does not address the ethics of inclusion as exploitation nor does it call upon me to reflect on my motivation. Consistent with this principle's emphasis on social equity in evaluation (Principle D-5), I would need to take special care to consider how the evaluation could benefit the consumers, not just how the consumers could benefit the evaluation.

WHAT I WOULD DO

Let's assume that I am still in conversation with the associate director. Despite the fact that her intensity makes me question my ability to change her mind, the Systematic Inquiry principle requires that I have such a discussion, exploring "the shortcomings and strengths both of the various evaluation questions and the various approaches that might be used" (American Evaluation Association, 2004, Principle A-2). I would take her reactivity to my mentioning service consumers as a signal that I do not fully appreciate the background and context of this evaluation. I need to know more about the culture of the organization, the priorities of the woman with whom I'm speaking, and her vision of how this evaluation can assist her in her role as associate director. I would delve deeper into both the evaluand and the evaluation.

Background and Context of the Evaluand

I would begin by responding to her last comment that the staff have "lived with this project most intimately over the past 2 years." I would affirm the importance of understanding what this experience has been like, and because I am detecting some power issues between us, I would do it in a way that positions her as the "expert" (e.g., "You're right that understanding the day-to-day impact of this project is very important. What have these past 2 years been like from your perspective?"). I would follow her lead and listen for both information and affect here. Has this been a stressful 2 years? If so, what does that say about her attitude toward this evaluation? For example, does she see it as adding more stress or as an opportunity to showcase the results of the project? Does she communicate any ownership of the project? Does she spontaneously mention consumer reactions to the project? I would listen for implied evaluation questions that might be important to address, and I would also try to ascertain her views about the coordination project itself, including her investment in it.

I would explain that a solid understanding of project context is important for valid inference in any evaluation (and, yes, I would use the phrase "valid inference" rather than paraphrase because I understand from her introduction of the terms "interview or survey" that she wants me to know that she understands research). I would ask how she would characterize the culture of this organization. I would let her talk without interruption as much as possible, probing on such matters as the nature of "working relationships" within OCPS, diversity of staff within the workforce, turnover of staff, and how change happens in this organization. Throughout her account, I am listening for any reference to recipients of services and noticing whether that comes from a deficit or strengths perspective. I recognize that I have already formed a snap judgment that she disrespects clients as whiners and complainers, and I need to listen for disconfirming information here.

I would try to get her story of the history of the relationships among the agencies involved. I assume that I've done my homework concerning public information about the agencies, their founding dates, missions, organizational structure, size, and so on, but I remain very much interested in her insider perspective on these groups, particularly if she has worked within this state system for a long time. (Note: If she has only recently arrived in the system, perhaps bringing the coordination project with her from another state, this presents a different but parallel set of questions, and it would require close inspection of similarities and differences between her prior context and the current one.) I am still listening for potentially relevant evaluation questions.

I would ask her to explain what she understands to be the scope of the working relationships of interest, and I would do so by asking for an example of what she envisions as a successful collaboration. I would listen carefully for success criteria implicitly embedded in her story and pay careful attention to how, if at all, she positions the consumer in this process. If she doesn't mention consumers, I make a mental note, but I don't pursue it at this time.

Background and Context of the Evaluation

It would be important to explore the history of evaluation within OCPS with respect to consumers in particular. The associate director asserts that this is not "the time or place for a study of client concerns," so I am curious whether such a study has been conducted in the past and, if so, with what consequences? Her comment that consumer surveys produce "a laundry list of complaints" suggests that data have been collected in the past that were not perceived as useful. I need to understand this history as well as what information she *has* previously found useful in her leadership role. That would lead me back to this evaluation. I would back up and try to ascertain in more detail its intended purpose.

To sort out the ethical issues more clearly, I want to know more about the influence she envisions this study having (Kirkhart, 2000). I would return to her role as an administrator and ask her to describe in her own words what she hopes to be able to learn from the evaluation and how she would use this information. I am assuming that she initiated the evaluation. If that's not the case, I would confirm whose idea it was to undertake the study, and I would seek to schedule a separate conversation with that person. I would probe the time frame within which these intended, results-based influences might unfold: What are the immediate needs for the information, and what uses does she envision flowing from that? How might the evaluation findings change the future operation of OCPS? I would also explore intended process-based influence (e.g., by asking how she expects staff to react to a request to participate in the evaluation). Is she hoping that the process of talking to a wide variety of agency representatives might change the system in a positive direction? Or that workers unhappy with the project would be mollified by having the opportunity to tell their story? To address unintended influences, I would ask if she has any concerns about undertaking this evaluation and whether she can envision any "bonus benefits" of doing so (i.e., positive influences that are beyond the overt purpose of the study itself) or ways in which it could "backfire" (i.e., negative impacts that might emerge).

Finally, I'd like to ascertain whom she sees as key stakeholders in this evaluation and work my way toward questions of potential interest to them. This project involves the coordination of several agencies; therefore, I would look for allies among the leadership of the involved organizations. Hopefully, there is a board or advisory council behind this project that has guided its implementation and could be consulted in shaping the evaluation. If she doesn't mention one, I would ask explicitly if there is a citizens' review board that is a stakeholder. I am listening for stakeholders she values who might show a greater interest in consumer inclusion than she does as a way to reintroduce this perspective. As a final strategy, I might refer to the mission statement of OCPS regarding the well-being of children and ask her how this evaluation could help her fulfill the mission of the office.

My Strategy

The intent of this line of questioning is twofold. First, I want to be sure that my understanding of context is solid so that I can avoid making unwarranted assumptions about consumer position. Inclusion of consumers, particularly those whose circumstances make them vulnerable by definition, is not to be taken lightly or ritualistically. I need to understand how consumers of services are positioned in relation to this project, including the extent to which the project is visible to them. To avoid the bias of my own value stance, I need to explore evidence that might disconfirm my assumption that consumer input is critical to obtaining valid answers to the questions at hand. Second, I am seeking to lay out a fair representation of the evaluation questions that are of most concern to the associate director and key stakeholders, hoping that this will permit me to move into a discussion of sources of information that would be necessary and appropriate to gain valid understandings. (I would be clear to focus on sources of information and *not* on data collection strategies. This is partly to "slow her down," because she already leaped to assumptions of method when consumers were mentioned, and partly to get around any reactivity she may have to a particular strategy, e.g., strong opposition to yet another consumer survey.) I would then reintroduce consumers as an important source of information for answering the questions as she has framed them, expressing concern about my ability to answer them well if we are missing that perspective.

The client requests "as much in-depth information from staff as you can [gather]," which suggests that she values thoroughness and does not desire a superficial study. I would reinforce this sentiment and argue that she would gain a false sense of the credibility and validity of the study if I were to follow her directive. I would lay out the questions that can legitimately be answered from staff and administrative perspectives only and those that require broader input. I would be explicit about exactly where consumers fit in the information-gathering picture. I would show the limitations of a narrow view and be clear about what could and could not be concluded from such an evaluation. I would be explicit in indicating how credible answers to her evaluation questions require exploration of multiple perspectives on this collaborative project. I would also "make it personal" by arguing that incomplete data put her at risk as an administrator, limiting her ability to make well-informed decisions that support the mission of her office.

I would probably conclude by suggesting that I put her ideas concerning evaluation questions in writing and draft some design options for discussion. I would recommend that we schedule another meeting to make sure we're "on the same page" before I produce a full proposal. I would explore her openness to my meeting with other key stakeholders to solicit evaluation questions of interest to them, but if she objects I would not push it at this point, knowing that I will build opportunities for such conversations into my evaluation design.

After listening respectfully to counterarguments, I would need to reflect carefully on what issues I consider open to negotiation. Because it appears that this client wants unambiguous control of the evaluation process up front, I must deal honestly with that restriction and not agree to anything that I would later try to finesse or get around. Consistent with the Respect for People principle, it is important that I be forthcoming about inclusion of the consumer perspective, and not try to sneak it into the design. Given my concerns about our differing value perspectives, I would also be careful to negotiate terms under which each party could dissolve the contract.

If the associate director declines to engage in further discussion and set another meeting, or if I cannot find the balance I seek by including consumers, it is not likely that I would continue to pursue this contract. My overarching ethical concerns remain. In this particular case and with this particular population, ignoring consumers of services legitimizes their position of powerlessness, sending exactly the wrong message to the OCPS system and producing incomplete and misleading findings. It is not in the best interests of the public good to proceed.

LESSONS LEARNED

If I could "turn back the clock" before the interaction described in this scenario, I would gather more background information on why the evaluation is being done and on the value perspectives of the client and key stakeholders. First, no mention is made of the rationale for the evaluation or what its anticipated or desired impact might be. Although I tried to address these issues in my conversation with the associate director, I should have done my homework more thoroughly in preparation. This information would set a broader context for the study from a systems perspective and flag potential covert agendas and possibilities of misuse that I should watch for (see the Integrity/ Honesty principle; American Evaluation Association, 2004, Principle C-5). Is the evaluation being conducted to support a reduction in the workforce? Is it part of a larger agenda to reduce state services to children and families? If consumers are not represented in this study, I would be especially concerned that the evaluation results could negatively impact services from the perspective of their lived experience.

Second, before a personal meeting with the associate director, I would try to discern the values of key stakeholders, noting in particular the extent to which there is consensus with respect to consumers' role and place in the system. To make the evaluation congruent with the nature of the project, I would seek to design the study collaboratively. I would try to create a mechanism (e.g., an advisory committee to the evaluation) for representing the full range of perspectives on the project, and I would request a group meeting as a setting for discussing issues of design. Whether in the group context or in an individual meeting with the associate director, I would ascertain others' perspectives *before* presenting my own. In the scenario, I expressed my opinions first.

The values clash that occurred probably could not have been avoided, but it certainly represents a good check on assumptions of presumed similarity within the helping professions; we are not all "on the same page" with respect to consumers. Given my background and values, I would surely question the absence of a consumer role in the study; "Where are the consumers in this evaluation?" is a question I have always explored from my earliest familiarity with *consumers* as an element in Scriven's (1991) Key Evaluation Checklist. It is a litmus test, to be sure, and sometimes it leads to a clash of perspectives, but it speaks volumes about the program, its staff and leadership, and the potential location of the evaluation itself. I would avoid an evaluation that takes a deficit perspective on program consumers or, by omission, communicates disrespect for their experience. I think it is important to have these concerns on the table early, so I don't see it as a bad thing that these values were revealed in our conversation. (And I would be sure to communicate this to the associate director with phrases like, "This is very helpful to me, because I want to understand your perspective," and so on.) But if she did not mention consumers as a stakeholder audience of interest to her, I still would have introduced the topic and we'd be off and running, probably in pretty much the same direction as the scenario depicts.

Cultural Competence

Although the case focuses our attention on consumers, cultural competence involves more than just primary inclusion of direct consumers in an evaluation (Hood, Hopson, & Frierson, 2005; Madison, 1992;

Thompson-Robinson, Hopson, & SenGupta, 2004). Cultural competence involves the knowledge, skills, and attitudes of persons doing evaluation, and it interacts with many of the Guiding Principles beyond its explicit mention in the Competence principle. A quick scan reveals the infusion of cultural competence throughout the Guiding Principles.

Knowledge

Cultural competence values historical knowledge, including relevant local history as well as understanding broader historical and political contexts (American Evaluation Association, 2004, Principle D-1). In this scenario, prerequisites to competent performance (Principle B-1) would include knowledge of child welfare policy and practices and of organizational development and management in order to address culture on both institutional and societal levels.

Skills

The accuracy and credibility called for by Systematic Inquiry (American Evaluation Association, 2004, Principle A-1) require skills in methods of investigation that are congruent with the culture of the evaluand and the communities that house it; in this case, the evaluand is collaborative and systemic, suggesting that the evaluation should be similarly positioned. Evaluators must be able to make transparent the culturally bound values and assumptions that shape the conceptualization of their work and the interpretation of findings (Principle A-3). Cultural competence includes the ability to listen openly and communicate respectfully with diverse audiences (Principle C-1) and to persist in difficult conversations about values (Principle C-4).

Attitudes

Cultural competence requires an attitude of respect for the evaluand and its diverse consumers, providers, and other stakeholders (American Evaluation Association, 2004, Principle D-6). It includes a commitment to fostering social equity (Principle D-5), designing an evaluation that gives *back* to those who participate in the evaluation—staff, supervisors and (it is hoped) consumers—and to the broader community and society (Principle E-5). It challenges evaluators to remain vigilant for possible unintended negative consequences of their work, such as unwittingly perpetuating institutional discrimination or leaving participants vulnerable to harm (Principle D-3), which is a definite possibility in this case. The culturally competent evaluator must engage in self-examination (Principle B-2) and be willing to be molded by what is revealed (Principle B-4). He or she must also be willing to disengage if conflicts of interest between client needs and the obligations of the Guiding Principles cannot be resolved (Principle E-4).

CONCLUSION

This exercise has been revealing. The Guiding Principles hold up well to the scrutiny of case application, and they achieve their goal of providing moral grounding for evaluation practice. They speak to specific points and present a framework for addressing crosscutting issues such as cultural competence. The case itself illustrates how easily culture can be overlooked. Evaluators face the challenge of seeing what's *not* presented and following relevant leads to bring missing pieces into clearer focus. It also offers a vivid illustration of the very human dynamics that shape the parameters of an evaluation, defining whose voices are amplified and whose are suppressed. Validity hangs in the balance.

REFERENCES

American Evaluation Association. (2004). *Guiding principles for evaluators* (rev.). Available at *www.eval.org/Publications/GuidingPrinciples.asp*.

Cronbach, L. J. (1988). Five perspectives on validity argument. In H. Wainer & H. I. Braun (Eds.), *Test validity* (pp. 3–17). Hillsdale, NJ: Erlbaum.

Hood, S., Hopson, R., & Frierson, H. (Eds.). (2005). *The role of culture and cultural context: A mandate for inclusion, the discovery of truth, and understanding in evaluative theory and practice.* Greenwich, CT: Information Age.

Kirkhart, K. E. (1995). Seeking multicultural validity: A postcard from the road. *Evaluation Practice, 16*(1), 1–12.

Kirkhart, K. E. (2000). Reconceptualizing evaluation use: An integrated theory of influence. In V. J. Caracelli & H. Preskill (Eds.), *The expanding scope of evaluation use* (New directions for program evaluation, no. 88, pp. 5–23). San Francisco: Jossey-Bass.

Kirkhart, K. E. (2005, April). *Cultural context and evaluative judgment.* Invited address presented at the annual meeting of the Eastern Evaluation Research Society, Absecon, NJ.

Madison, A. (1992). Primary inclusion of culturally diverse minority program participants in the evaluation process. In A. Madison (Ed.), *Minority issues in program evaluation* (New directions for program evaluation, no. 53, pp. 35–43). San Francisco: Jossey-Bass.

Messick, S. (1980). Test validity and the ethics of assessment. *American Psychologist, 35,* 1012–1027.

Messick, S. (1995). Validity of psychological assessment: Validation of inferences from persons' responses and performances as scientific inquiry into score meaning. *American Psychologist, 50,* 741–749.

National Association of Social Workers. (2001). *NASW standards for cultural competence in social work practice.* Available at *www.socialworkers.org/sections/credentials/cultural_comp.asp.*

Ridley, C. R., Mendoza, D. W., Kanitz, B. E., Angermeier, L., & Zenk, R. (1994). Cultural sensitivity in multicultural counseling: A perceptual schema model. *Journal of Counseling Psychology, 41,* 125–136.

Scriven, M. (1991). *Evaluation thesaurus* (4th ed.). Newbury Park, CA: Sage.

Thompson-Robinson, M., Hopson, R., & SenGupta, S. (Eds.). (2004). *In search of cultural competence in evaluation: Toward principles and practices* (New directions for evaluation, no. 102). San Francisco: Jossey-Bass.

Whose Evaluation Is It, Anyway?

David M. Chavis

In my view, this case involves balancing personal values with professional standards for systematic inquiry. Often we are faced with the challenge of proposing or planning evaluations that can provide technically adequate information despite their limitations but that might not be conducted in a manner consistent with our values. The primary ethical question is whether the study of the coordination project is seriously limited by the absence of a consumer component. The potential client has asked the evaluator to determine "the extent to which the project has enhanced working relationships among the agencies involved." Some evaluators will believe that having consumer input is essential for a credible evaluation of this type. Others, including myself, believe that a technically sound investigation of agency relationships can be done without consumer input. We probably would all agree that a more thorough evaluation would include consumer perceptions and assess how agency relationships affect the quality of services. However, that "better evaluation" is not what is being requested. The question the evaluator has to ponder is whether requiring consumer input is a personal value or a methodological necessity, and is it consistent with professional ethics?

WHAT CAN WE LEARN FROM THE GUIDING PRINCIPLES?

The Guiding Principles for Evaluators point to areas for evaluators to consider in managing their professional behavior. The application of the first two Guiding Principles—Systematic Inquiry and Competence—challenges the evaluator to determine what sources of information are essential to competently conduct systematic inquiry into the questions presented by the client. The evaluator has to determine whether the Guiding Principles are being addressed in an acceptable manner. It is important for the evaluator to identify his or her own acceptable levels and to identify appropriate practices related to these principles.

If the evaluator believes that consumer input is essential to produce a quality evaluation in this case, then the evaluator is compelled to take action. On the other hand, if consumer input is a personal value based on the evaluator's sense of social justice or other issues not related to methodological quality and technical matters, I think the evaluator's responsibilities are different, and another approach is called for.

Thus, if the evaluator believes that the absence of consumer input would lead to "misleading evaluative information or conclusions," according to the Integrity/Honesty principle, the evaluator has "the responsibility to communicate their concerns and the reasons for them" (American Evaluation Association, 2004, Principle C-6). The Guiding Principles encourage evaluators to decline conducting a study if these concerns cannot be adequately addressed. In this way, the integrity and honesty of the evaluation are protected.

At other times, evaluators may find themselves in situations that challenge their sense of social justice or equality, even though a proposed design might be satisfactory on conventional technical grounds. They may believe that certain improvements in the evaluation's design (e.g., including consumer input) would enhance the evaluation and make it more worthwhile. In the scenario, for example, the evaluator needs to decide whether data from consumers are crucial for an adequate evaluation in terms of his or her own "guiding principles" and personal standards. If they are seen as crucial, then I believe that the evaluator is ethically obligated not to accept this assignment or contract if his or her best efforts to persuade the potential client do not succeed.

WHAT IS NOT COVERED BY THE GUIDING PRINCIPLES?

The Guiding Principles do not fully address the prerogative of clients to ensure that the evaluation meets their needs and to adjust the scope of the work as they see fit within ethical and technical boundaries. Clients have every right, and in many cases the obligation to their own organization, to reduce the scope or focus of the evaluation as they deem appropriate.

I have found myself in this situation many times. I can get very excited about the possibilities of answering additional questions or examining questions deeper or further than the client may have originally envisioned. I have also learned that this is often a very short-sighted view of the evaluation process. In my personal practice and as part of our overall organizational culture, meeting and exceeding client expectations is a core value that helps us achieve excellence in our work. I have found that I can simultaneously be client driven and practice evaluation ethically. To do this requires not only an understanding of my own ethics and values but also that I consider the motivation and values of my client. Most of all it requires the assumption of respect for a client's decision-making authority and intentions, unless proven otherwise. Although the Guiding Principles do address the general issue of respect for all stakeholders (e.g., respondents), the need for particular respect for the evaluator's *clients* is not as clearly delineated.

Underlying this case is the assumption that the associate director does not want information from consumers. Indeed, evaluators often believe that we value truth more than our clients. But in situations like the coordination project, we need to look for the truth in what the client or others are saying. Perhaps the associate director has had past experience with your evaluation work or with studies conducted by another evaluator. That experience may have led to her opinion about consumer input. Or she may have had no experience with evaluations that have provided useful information about consumer perspectives. Maybe she wants to focus the evaluation somewhat narrowly in order to get the most for her agency's limited money. These are important possibilities to explore.

WHAT CAN AN EVALUATOR DO?

In many ways, producing a successful evaluation is all about building good relationships as part of a learning process. If I were the evaluator in this situation, I would accept the assignment as an ethically and technically acceptable evaluation plan, provided that what is being requested could be developed and implemented with the resources that were available. I would use my interactions with the associate director in this evaluation as an opportunity to better understand her concerns over consumer input. I would build a relationship based on mutual trust and respect. It would be essential that the final product of this assignment demonstrate that both positive and negative information can result in useful recommendations. If the associate director truly fears receiving negative feedback from consumers, having constructive and comfortable discussions of critical information *now* would make it easier to incorporate consumer views into future evaluation efforts.

Before submission of the final report, I would meet with the associate director to reflect on the study's findings. We generally require this in all of our evaluation contracts. At that time, we would discuss the evaluation's results, lessons learned, implications for action, and future learning or evaluation opportunities. At this point, it may be appropriate to raise the question of the system's readiness to explore the impact of the intervention on consumers. If I have been able to conserve resources during the evaluation (i.e., if I have money left in the evaluation budget), this might increase the likelihood of such a follow-up study occurring, because having adequate funds to address the associate director's questions was a concern of hers. This assumes, of course, that I have succeeded in establishing a strong relationship with my client based on respect and mutual learning, not just compatible personalities. Such a bond is conducive to the ethical practice of evaluation not only in the case of the coordination project but in other situations as well.

A relationship with leadership based on learning is needed to generate an organizational culture change in which evaluation is used to improve capacity (e.g., knowledge and skills). This begins with the evaluator, through relationship development, discovering what challenges or needs the associate director is facing and how evaluation might help address them. Often, addressing these issues may not be an explicit part of my contract but something I try to make happen nonetheless. Perhaps it is a need for immediate information on program success, or appropriately sharing information on misconceptions about the program, that is causing tensions. In one evaluation I conducted, it was staff concerns about dwindling client participation that led to collecting information from consumers.

Demonstrating the practical value of evaluation is one of the most important tasks for an evaluator looking to build a relationship based on learning that can make a difference. In this sense, evaluators must be opportunists, helping clients use findings to enhance their knowledge, problem-solving capacity, and legitimate interests.

REFERENCE

American Evaluation Association. (2004). *Guiding principles for evaluators* (rev.). Available at *www.eval.org/Publications/GuidingPrinciples.asp*.

■ ■ ■ ■

WHAT IF . . . ?

. . . *a recent feature article in a local newspaper had reported anecdotal data indicating that parents and foster families were pleased with how the coordination project was working?*

. . . *the associate director has a national reputation as an expert on interagency collaboration and is viewed as a "rising star" within the statewide human services hierarchy?*

. . . *the associate director argues that a study of consumer perceptions would be much more valuable if it were conducted after an evaluation of the staff's experiences with the coordination project?*

FINAL THOUGHTS

The Coordination Project

In characterizing the results of a study of evaluators' views of ethical issues, Morris and Jacobs (2000) noted that "to those who would like to see evaluators 'speak with one voice' on ethical matters . . . the bad news is that one voice does not exist" (p. 402). Much the same can be said when reflecting on the analyses of Kirkhart and Chavis. The starting point for both commentators is roughly the same: Is it possible to conduct a valid, methodologically sound evaluation of the coordination project—one that satisfies the Guiding Principles for Evaluators—without including consumer perspectives? It is their *answers* to this question that markedly differ.

Chavis is optimistic that a respectable study can be performed; Kirkhart is not. Chavis emphasizes the right of the evaluation client to determine the focus of the research. Although he believes that the evaluation might be *improved* by the incorporation of a consumer component, he does not see such a component as essential to the investigation. Perceiving it as essential would, in Chavis's opinion, be a product of the evaluator's *personal values* being applied to the situation. The evaluator could certainly choose to walk away from the proposed study if this were the case, but it would be personal values, rather than the Guiding Principles, that are driving the decision.

Put simply, Kirkhart disagrees. Given the nature of the coordination project, she believes that the Guiding Principles require that consumer perspectives be gathered as part of the evaluation. She presents her argument in great detail and links her analysis to the evaluator's responsibility for designing a study that takes into account the culture of the system being researched, a system that includes, at the very least, both service providers *and* consumers. Kirkhart acknowledges that her own background and values are likely contributors to her response to the case, but it is the Guiding Principles that she sees as providing the foundation for her analysis.

So, who is right? Do the Guiding Principles require the consumer-inclusive approach that Kirkhart advocates, or do they leave room, in this instance, for a client-driven evaluation that omits consumer views? Is this just a vivid example of how the abstract quality of professional standards can result in situations in which, as Rossi (1995) puts it, "members will be able to claim conformity [to such standards] no matter what they do" (p. 59)? What verdict do you see the Guiding Principles rendering on The Coordination Project case?

REFERENCES

Morris, M., & Jacobs, L. R. (2000). You got a problem with that? Exploring evaluators' disagreements about ethics. *Evaluation Review, 24,* 384–406.

Rossi, P. H. (1995). Doing good and getting it right. In W. R. Shadish, D. L. Newman, M. A. Scheirer, & C. Wye (Eds.), *Guiding principles for evaluators* (New directions for program evaluation, no. 66, pp. 55–59). San Francisco: Jossey-Bass.

Just Say No?

The school system for which you serve as an internal evaluator has recently revised its curriculum to incorporate concepts from the "intelligent design" literature into selected science courses at various grade levels. Conventional evolutionary theory continues to be taught in these courses, but it is now presented as just one of several ways of explaining how organisms evolve that students can choose from in the marketplace of ideas. The superintendent wants you to evaluate the impact of this curriculum revision on students' knowledge of, and attitudes toward, conventional evolutionary theory, concepts of intelligent design, and the general nature of scientific inquiry.

Your initial reaction to this assignment can best be described as "conflicted." It is your firm belief that the topic of intelligent design does *not* belong in science courses. You have not come to this conclusion lightly. You have reviewed with care the arguments pro and con on the issue, and the verdict of the scientific community seems virtually unanimous: Science courses are not the place where intelligent design should be taught, given that this school of thought operates outside of the rules of hypothesis testing, evidence, and proof that govern scientific inquiry. Thus, to evaluate the impact of intelligent design in science courses bestows legitimacy, implicitly if not explicitly, on an educational practice that is fundamentally ill-conceived. Indeed, as an evaluator you see yourself as a member of the scientific community, and you do not wish your work to contribute to a climate in which intelligent design is seen as simply another intervention in the field of education whose effects need to be investigated. Such an outcome would, in your mind, shift attention away from the core problem that intelligent design's presence in science courses represents. To borrow a metaphor from the legal system, attention would be focused on the "fruit of the poisoned tree" rather than on the tree itself.

On the other hand, your resistance to evaluating this curriculum revision is making you feel a bit like those pharmacists who refuse to fill prescriptions for medications they object to on religious grounds—and you don't like that feeling. The community's democratically elected school board supports the intelligent design initiative, and surveys indicate a high level of support for the idea in the community as a whole. Don't these stakeholders have a right to expect that data will be gathered about the curriculum revision? Couldn't such data lead to a more informed discussion of the appropriateness of intelligent design in science courses? If you balk at conducting the evaluation, could you be accused of displaying the same sort of nonscientific attitude that, in your view, intelligent design reflects?

The superintendent is meeting with you tomorrow morning to discuss the evaluation. What are you going to say to her?

QUESTIONS TO CONSIDER

1. In what ways, if any, are the Guiding Principles for Evaluators relevant to this case?

2. Is the pharmacist analogy an appropriate one to apply here? Why or why not?

3. Would it make a difference if you were the sole internal evaluator working in the school system versus being one member of a team of internal evaluators? What if there were funds available to hire an external evaluator for this project? Would you lobby for the superintendent to do that?

4. Would refusing to conduct the evaluation represent an empty, symbolic gesture that does more harm than good to the reputation of the school system's evaluation unit?

5. Is having more data about a program always better than having fewer data?

6. What if your input as an evaluator had been solicited during the stage at which the intelligent design curriculum revision was being planned? What would have been your response?

CHAPTER THREE

Designing the Evaluation

The Damp Parade?

In the public school system where you serve as director of program evaluation, a new superintendent is on the scene. His commitment to evaluation is significantly greater than his predecessor's, as can be seen in his response to a peer-mentoring program currently being offered in a subset of middle schools and high schools throughout the city. The program was initiated last year in collaboration with a prestigious local community services agency (CSA) that specializes in prevention-oriented interventions focused on youth. At that time, funds were not available to evaluate the program, but with the new superintendent's arrival a few months ago, the situation has changed. He would like you to conduct an impact evaluation of the program and is willing to provide resources for that purpose.

For the past several weeks, you have been meeting with the CSA professionals (a PhD psychologist and two MSWs) who developed the peer-mentoring program and oversee its implementation in the schools. The early meetings went well, with the group reaching consensus on a moderately strong quasi-experimental design to assess impact. You are now in the midst of discussing *how* to measure the program's outcomes, and significant disagreement has emerged. The CSA representatives recommend using a variety of survey and interview instruments that they have employed in several other school districts around the state where the agency's peer mentoring program has been adopted. You have reviewed these measures and are unimpressed by their technical adequacy. Indeed, in many respects they seem to represent little more than customer satisfaction measures. Not surprisingly, no systematic data exist on the instruments' reliability or validity. There is only the limited face validity of the items themselves. You have also noted with interest that the results generated by these measures appear in brochures and other printed materials that the CSA provides to school districts that are considering adopting the program.

In your view, a more rigorous approach to measurement is called for. You want to develop a stronger set of survey and interview measures and perhaps make use of relevant organizational records (e.g., grades) as well. The CSA representatives are not thrilled with your suggestions, which they characterize as "methodological overkill." They assert that peer-mentoring programs have gained acceptance in school systems across the country and that the CSA's measures are well suited to what should be a *formative* impact evaluation rather than a *summative* one.

Following the meeting in which these differences of opinion surfaced, you have the opportunity to meet one on one with the superintendent, with whom you have a direct reporting relationship. You share your concerns with him and show him CSA's survey and interview measures. After briefly reviewing them, the superintendent hands the copies back to you and comments that "most of these items look pretty reasonable to me, but you're the expert here. Do what you think is best, but keep in mind that we don't need to have a bullet-proof, gold-standard, methodologically pristine type of study here. I just want to make sure that we gather some defensible data about the program so that we can tell the Board of Education that what we spend on peer mentoring isn't just money flushed down the toilet."

Your conversation with the superintendent has only made you queasier about this whole situation. You suspect that the CSA wants a weak evaluation to protect its interests, whereas the superintendent's main concern seems to be one of keeping the Board of Education off his back. But he's leaving the decision about how to proceed up to you.

You begin to wonder, "How much rain am I justified in dumping on this parade?"

Everybody Talks about the Weather . . .

Melvin M. Mark

Okay, let me see if I've got this right. You find yourself in a bit of a quandary. There's a new superintendent in the school district where you work. With his encouragement, you've been planning an impact evaluation of a school-based peer-mentoring program. Together with the CSA that developed and now implements the program, you agreed on a "moderately strong quasi-experimental design." But then you ran into disagreement with the CSA about the measures to use in the evaluation. They want to employ more consumer satisfaction-type measures, and you don't think these are adequate. The superintendent, after initially supporting the idea of doing the evaluation, seems to be siding with the CSA. He even told you that you don't need—what was it?—a "gold-standard, methodologically pristine" evaluation. Instead, he just wants some defensible data to show the Board of Education that the program isn't a waste of money. All of this makes you wonder. What you're wondering, I'm guessing, is not only about how to deal with this particular evaluation but also what the future holds for you as director of program evaluation.

So here you are, asking me for advice. That alone may be a sign of how desperate you are! I probably should be getting ready for my conference presentation later this afternoon. But what are conferences for, if not to sit and converse with friends and colleagues? If we had more time, I'd probably ask you a bunch of questions and try to talk this through back and forth. For the time being, though, let me just put some thoughts on the table, and we can discuss them later if you'd like. In a way this might more make sense. After all, if you have an ethical challenge, it probably deserves the contemplation of more than one sitting.

TO BEGIN, A WARNING

You ended your description of the situation by asking, "How much rain am I justified in dumping on this parade?" Well, you know me. I love to take a good metaphor and carry it to excess, so expect a veritable flood!

But seriously, your question reminds me of the old expression "Everybody talks about the weather, but nobody does anything about it." Maybe this is a case where you should try to do something about the upcoming stormy conditions. Then if you find you can't affect the weather, you might want to get an umbrella or build a shelter or, at the extreme, move to drier ground. First, though, I think you should make sure that you have an accurate forecast before you decide how to act. And, again, regardless of the forecast, you should consider whether you can influence the odds of rain before you start calling for a downpour at parade time.

FIRST STEP: GET A MORE CERTAIN FORECAST

Let me explain why I believe you need to begin by getting a better forecast. First, you mentioned that the superintendent wants you to conduct an impact evaluation. You also indicated that you and the CSA have agreed on a "moderately strong quasi-experimental design." Maybe we can come back to the details of the design later because there seem to be interesting possibilities. For example, it sounds like some schools will receive the program while others will not, thus allowing you to measure both preprogram cohorts and postintervention cohorts on certain outcome variables. I'm reminded of what Campbell and Stanley (1966) called a "patched-up" design. In various ways, then, you might be able to do even better than a "moderately strong" design. But, at the moment, let's set aside design issues and stick with the possible ethical challenge you're facing.

One of the things I'm trying to figure out is how the decision to have a quasi-experimental impact evaluation fits with the use of satisfaction measures only. If all the superintendent wants is a measure of customer satisfaction, why would he have talked about an impact evaluation? And why would there be any motivation to use a quasi-experimental design? Wouldn't it be easier just to give out the satisfaction measure to participants at the end of the program? And I'm assuming that you're not talking about the common kind of consumer satisfaction measure that simply asks people to indicate their satisfaction with various attributes of the program, because items like that wouldn't seem to work well in a comparison group where students didn't participate in the program.

Second, the CSA people indicated that they're thinking about a formative evaluation rather than a summative one. If that's the case, would it have made sense for them to agree to a quasi-experimental design and a moderately strong one at that? Couldn't you get the same formative benefits without the extra time and expense your quasi-experimental design is likely to require? And if the CSA folks are thinking in terms of formative evaluation, why are they talking about a formative *impact* evaluation? I know different people use phrases like "impact evaluation" in different ways, but even so I'm having trouble making sense of all this. Heck, if the CSA people are serious about conducting a good formative evaluation, would satisfaction-type data alone buy enough learning to justify the effort?

Finally, consider the superintendent's reference to "defensible data" and to convincing the Board of Education. These notions probably suggest a more summative evaluation. If so, how does the idea of convincing the board fit with the CSA representatives suggesting that the evaluation is more formative? And are the kinds of satisfaction measures that worry you likely to be persuasive to the board anyway? Sorry to be showering you with so many questions, but I'm in a bit of a fog trying to understand how everything fits together.

In short, what all of this adds up to is that all of this doesn't seem to add up, at least to me. So, before you get too far into raining on the parade, I think you need to check your forecast. Is it really overcast, with a 90% chance of public relations masquerading as evaluation? Or might the forecast be sunnier than you think?

On the issue of how cloudy it is, I'd counsel you to be careful not to jump too quickly to the conclusion that the superintendent's motives are bad. After all, he did say that "you're the expert" and that you should "do what you think is best." Maybe he's just trying to snow you, but it doesn't necessarily sound to me like he's trying to subvert the evaluation. Assuming that the superintendent has negative intentions could get you in a needless mud-throwing contest, and that probably isn't the most ethical approach!

WAS A PAST—OR CURRENT—EVALUATOR A DRIP?

Let's think about what else might have led the superintendent to say what he did. We all know that some evaluators push for a methodological gold standard, even when this may not make sense in light of the information needs of relevant stakeholders. For example, the evaluator might implement a methodologically sophisticated design that sounds good to method geeks like us but fails to provide usable findings in a timely fashion. It's possible that your new superintendent has had experience with evaluators who ignored practical constraints, or who were driven by a dogmatic view of method choices, or who were not really responsive to stakeholders' needs. So the superintendent might be influenced by these kinds of concerns without explicitly accusing you of doing the same thing. He may not want to do your job, but he also may not yet be confident that you'll do it well.

Indeed, depending on what you had suggested—and forgive me for raising the possibility—you might have set off alarm bells, or should I say storm warnings, in the superintendent's mind. You mentioned that you were thinking about using grades and other information from organizational records. Before you do this, I'd want to be sure that there's a sound logic model or program theory indicating that improved grades, or changes in the other kinds of archival outcomes you might have access to, are a plausible consequence of this program. Even if theory does suggest such effects, is it plausible to expect them given that the program was just implemented last year? Might the superintendent have inferred that you were planning an evaluation that would be technically impressive, but would set up criteria or standards of merit that the new program couldn't reasonably hope to achieve?

Let's explore the implications here. Imagine that no sensible program theory would claim that the program should affect grades. Also imagine that, not surprisingly, you end up with an evaluation report showing that the program doesn't affect grades. In today's climate of No Child Left Behind and high-stakes testing, let's make it even more intense: Suppose you find the program doesn't increase test scores. This would put the program and the superintendent in something of a bind. If the superintendent tells the Board of Education that the program doesn't affect test scores—even if it wasn't set up to do that— then the board may wonder whether they should support the program. Indeed, the fact that the expert evaluation team examined test scores might suggest to board members that an effect on grades was expected. After all, why else look at them? You know how Patton (1997) and others have been talking about process use, where the dynamics of being involved in an evaluation, rather than the findings themselves, leads to some form of use? Well, in a recent chapter Mills and I (Mark & Mills, 2007) suggest generalizing this idea and talking about "procedural influence." The notion here is that procedural aspects of an evaluation (like what gets measured) can influence attitudes and actions (like what outcomes the board thinks the program should affect). The way people talk about process evaluation seems to limit its effects to those individuals directly involved in the evaluation process. Mills and I suggest that evaluation procedures can have wider consequences, influencing even those who weren't directly involved in the evaluation. Couldn't it be unfair to the program, and to the clients that it serves, if you encourage the Board of Education to think in terms of test scores as an expected outcome, if that's not what the program was designed to accomplish? What if the program then is eliminated in spite of its having other beneficial effects for which it was intended? What would the Guiding Principle of Responsibilities for General and Public Welfare say about this?

Now, let's imagine again that you do the evaluation and, to no one's surprise, you don't find an effect on test scores. This time, however, assume that the superintendent decides not to report this part of the evaluation to the board. Then there'd be a concern about whether everybody is being intellectually honest or whether the superintendent is censoring the evaluation. This could end up being a dark cloud over the new superintendent's entire administration.

An evaluation that overreaches in terms of the outcomes it measures, by which I mean an evaluation that measures outcomes that the program is not intended to affect, that no plausible program theory has suggested it should affect, and that stakeholders have not identified as a valued potential outcome of the program, could easily lead to undesirable consequences. I'll admit that there may be other ways to reduce that risk. But it could result in a hailstorm, not just heavy rain, if your evaluation treats grades and test scores as program outcomes when it shouldn't. And my main point is that it's premature to get pessimistic about the superintendent. He could have valid reasons for putting the brakes on an overly ambitious evaluation that might hold the program to the wrong criteria of merit. Bob Dylan sang, "You don't have to be a weatherman to know which way the wind's blowing." If your evaluation makes the board pay attention to grades or test scores or other archival information when these aren't the appropriate criteria for judging the program, the superintendent might conclude that he didn't have to be an evaluator to know which way your evaluation plans were blowing.

Now I'll back up for a second. I've been ranting a bit without even asking you if grades and test scores actually make sense as outcomes, given the program's objectives, the program theory, and so on. Come to think of it, I suppose that improving academic achievement could be the main point of the peer-mentoring program. Still, *even if* grades and test scores are sensible outcome measures, I'd probably ask whether the program is mature enough to be held responsible for affecting them within the timeline of the evaluation. As you know, people who talk about "program stage" as a guide to evaluation design typically suggest a period of formative evaluation before moving to summative evaluation. You, the CSA, the superintendent, and perhaps others need to ask whether the program is sufficiently developed for a summative evaluation.

Even if test grades or other archival data are appropriate, I would also ask some technical questions, such as whether you'll have adequate statistical power (especially with nested data) to be confident that the evaluation would detect an effect if one is there. Technical considerations like this can determine whether an evaluation might inadvertently do harm, and that seems like a pretty important ethical matter, doesn't it?

LINKS TO THE GUIDING PRINCIPLES

So, where are we? Well, before you start precipitating on anyone's parade, my recommendation is that you double-check your forecast. To some extent, all this means is going back to common procedures that evaluators use and indeed to the Guiding Principles for Evaluators (American Evaluation Association, 2004). A lot of what I have been talking about falls under the Systematic Inquiry principle, which deals with exploring strengths and weaknesses of evaluation questions and approaches as well as the principle of Integrity/Honesty, which focuses on honest negotiation with clients and stakeholders about things such as the evaluation methods and their limits and the likely uses of the resulting data. Similarly, the Program Evaluation Standards (Joint Committee on Standards for Educational Evaluation, 1994) call for ensuring that evaluation information is responsive to the needs of clients and other relevant stakeholders. What I'm suggesting is that, if you back up a little and rechart your course for planning the evaluation's focus and methods, and do so in a way that ensures you are responsive to our professional standards, you'll discover whether you really do have an ethical challenge. You might even avoid an ethical problem that otherwise would occur. At that point, if the forecast is still nasty, then you can try to do something about the weather.

ADDING SOME SUNSHINE TO YOUR LONG-TERM WEATHER PATTERNS

As director of program evaluation, you probably are responsible for keeping "Stormy Weather" from becoming the theme song of your department for years to come. One possible limitation of the Guiding Principles (and the Program Evaluation Standards) is that they focus on the way evaluators do an *individual* study. However, I think a case can be made that some ethical challenges go beyond the single evaluation. Think about your responsibility for the long-term role that evaluation can play—or not play—within your school system. For somebody like you, the educative function that Cronbach and others have talked about isn't just about a single evaluation project but about evaluation in general (Cronbach et al., 1980).

You have a new superintendent who seems interested in evaluation. At least he's provided you with support for evaluating this peer-mentoring program. And he also appears committed to *using* evaluation. After all, he's talking about taking evaluation results to the board. Not every superintendent blows onto the scene and right away starts discussing evaluation use in this fashion with the director of evaluation. It looks as though you may well be in the enviable position of working with, and, in the best sense of the word, educating the new superintendent about evaluation.

You can help make sure that he understands the benefits and limits of evaluation. You can talk about the different purposes of evaluation, including more summative and more formative ones. You can try to reach agreement about when each purpose is more appropriate for the school district. You can discuss the kinds of trade-offs one typically faces when planning an evaluation. You can address evaluation use and misuse. You can also talk about the professional guidelines that exist and about your own commitment to following them. And you can reflect on how adherence to those guidelines limits your ability to contribute to a public relations function when the data don't justify it. I don't want to shower you with too much at once, but to return to your rain metaphor, you're in the springtime of your relationship with the superintendent. And that's the season, especially if rain is anticipated, when it's best to plan and plant your garden.

I'm not saying that you should attempt to do all this education right now. Still, discussion of the peer-mentoring program gives you an excellent opportunity to begin addressing some of these educational opportunities. You can work through the details of this evaluation in a way that helps lay the groundwork for the future. Again, however, the educative function that you serve should not be a one-time deal. It's not so much about short-term weather as it is about long-term climate change.

USE AND MISUSE

The circumstances you're facing are linked to the issue of evaluation use and misuse. It sounds like what you are really worried about is that you might do an evaluation that is misused. In particular, it seems your fear is that, if you do an evaluation focusing on satisfaction data, it would be used to make a claim about the program's effectiveness, merit, and worth, even though the evaluation data wouldn't truly justify such a claim. From this perspective, then, the core ethical challenge in this case is the possibility of misuse.

Once again, the Guiding Principles are relevant. The Integrity/Honesty principle states that "evaluators should not misrepresent their procedures, data or findings" (American Evaluation Association, 2004, Principle C-5). That's not what is distressing you. But this principle goes on to say "within reasonable limits, they [the evaluators] should attempt to prevent or correct misuse of their work by others" (Principle C-5). If "misleading evaluative information or conclusions" (Principle C-6) are likely to result, the evaluator has a responsibility to explain his or her concerns. Then, if misuse is still likely, "the evaluator should decline to conduct the evaluation" (Principle C-6). This principle further states that if it isn't feasible to decline the evaluation—which may well apply to your situation; you're not a private consultant, after all—then the "evaluator should consult colleagues or relevant stakeholders about other proper ways to proceed" (Principle C-6). I guess that's what you're doing now, proactively consulting with colleagues. I think many ethical guidelines, such as those of the American Psychological Association, likewise refer to consultation with colleagues when one is faced with an ethical challenge. So you've "done good" in this regard, with the possible exception of your choice of whom to consult!

Consultation is an important step. And I hope that this conversation and others help you find a way to avoid misuse. But what if the worst-case scenario comes true, and you are certain that misuse will occur? The Integrity/Honesty principle gives examples of ways to proceed if your conversations with clients don't alleviate concerns about the possibility of misuse. One is to have discussions at a higher level, which in your situation would probably mean the Board of Education.

Other options are to include a minority report or "dissenting cover letter or appendix" (American Evaluation Association, 2004, Principle C-6) or to refuse to sign the final report.

Of course, if it gets this far, you may need to make sure that you have some kind of cover to protect you from whatever falls from the sky. And if you see *really* nasty weather coming, you might have to start looking for shelter from the storm, perhaps even a new job (the metaphorical "higher ground"). This possibility, however, raises an ethical and moral dilemma that I think the Guiding Principles do not adequately address: conflicts between ethical standards for evaluation and *other* moral responsibilities you may have. For example, I'm not sure I'd want you to take an ethical hard line about this evaluation, if it means that you would end up living on the street with those beautiful kids of yours. You also would have to think about the consequences of your actions for the people who work for you in the evaluation unit. Would they be put at risk if you refused to do the evaluation or raised a stink with the board? Of course, that's the real core of ethical challenges, isn't it, when ethical principles are in conflict?

Thinking about possible costs for your family and others makes it even clearer how crucial it is that you do whatever you can to *prevent* misuse from happening rather than stirring up a storm after the fact. And that takes us back to the educative function we've already talked about and to the even earlier step of making sure you have an adequate forecast about the likelihood of misuse.

AN OPTION WE HAVE MIST?

It occurs to me that there may be another way out of this challenging situation. Have you looked at existing evidence on the effects of peer-mentoring programs like this one? I'm wondering if there might even be a meta-analysis summarizing previous evaluations. If there is a substantial prior literature demonstrating that this kind of program generally works, that information alone might be enough to take to the Board of Education, satisfying the superintendent's concern, at least in the short term. This approach would especially make sense if similar programs have been shown to be effective in school systems like yours or if a meta-analysis shows that the effects of peer-mentoring programs are relatively robust and occur in a wide range of situations.

If there is a strong and persuasive body of prior evaluations indicating that programs like this are typically effective—whether from a

meta-analysis or not—you might see if this suffices for the superintendent and the board for the time being. Indeed, then you could legitimately think of the current evaluation of your school system's peer-
mentoring program as more formative than summative. Indeed, if a
meta-analysis exists, it might even be helpful in terms of formative
evaluation. Some meta-analyses report larger effects when a program
is implemented in certain ways. For example, I think that in adult
mentoring programs, greater impacts are observed when the intervention includes high-quality training about mentoring along with some
other characteristics. If there's evidence like this in an existing meta-
analysis, one part of your formative evaluation might be to see how
well your program measures up in terms of having the program components that have proved beneficial elsewhere.

Let's imagine that you can do this; that is, assume that you can
rely on evaluative evidence from elsewhere to satisfy your stakeholder's short-term concerns about whether (or should I say
"weather"?) it's reasonable to invest in the peer-mentoring program.
Then you could work, in the long term, on all of the educative issues
we've talked about without this work having to take place in the heat
of the moment around the evaluation of this particular program. You
also could use this opportunity to collaborate with the superintendent,
the CSA, maybe even somebody from the Board of Education, and
whatever other stakeholders make sense in thinking about what *series*
of evaluative activities are appropriate for the peer-mentoring program. This should provide a good context for ongoing education of all
constituencies.

I have a caveat. Something you said makes me doubtful about
whether a great deal of solid, convincing evidence exists showing that
peer-mentoring programs of this particular type are effective. If I heard
you correctly, you said that the CSA representatives argued that you
didn't need a summative evaluation because these kind of programs
had "gained acceptance" in school systems across the country. Certainly, the experience of the DARE evaluations demonstrates that gain-
ing acceptance, in the sense of getting implemented within scores of
schools, doesn't necessarily imply program effectiveness. Anyway, my
guess is that, if there already were numerous summative evaluations
showing that this peer-mentoring program works, the CSA would
have said so. However, I'm just drawing an inference here. So you
should make sure that you know what the existing evaluations of this
program, or very similar ones, are saying. If a meta-analysis is out
there, it might contain strong enough evidence pertaining to *this kind*

of peer-mentoring program, even if there haven't been many summative evaluations of this *specific program*. If that is the case, then, as I already mentioned, you could delay your own summative evaluation for a while and instead focus on a formative project now.

GOODBYE, AND MAY THE WIND BE AT YOUR BACK

Hey, I've gotta run. Sorry I was spouting off so much, but your question unleashed a veritable deluge of thoughts. I hope some of my verbal downpour helps you to think through this challenge. And let me suggest a theme song for the soundtrack of this part of your life. Remember that old Creedence Clearwater Revival tune "Who'll Stop the Rain?"? It could be you.

REFERENCES

American Evaluation Association. (2004). *Guiding principles for evaluators* (rev.). Available at *www.eval.org/Publications/GuidingPrinciples.asp*.

Campbell, D. T., & Stanley, J. C. (1966). *Experimental and quasi-experimental designs for research*. Chicago: Rand McNally.

Cronbach, L. J., Ambron, S. R., Dornbusch, S. M., Hess, R. D., Hornik, R. C., Phillips, D. C., et al. (1980). *Toward reform of program evaluation*. San Francisco: Jossey-Bass.

Joint Committee on Standards for Educational Evaluation. (1994). *The program evaluation standards: How to assess evaluations of educational programs* (2nd ed.). Thousand Oaks, CA: Sage.

Mark, M. M., & Mills, J. (2007). The use of experiments and quasi-experiments in decision making. In G. Marcöl (Ed.), *Handbook of decision making* (pp. 459–482). New York: Marcel Dekker.

Patton, M. Q. (1997). *Utilization-focused evaluation: The new century text* (3rd ed.). Thousand Oaks, CA: Sage.

No Rain Today

Gail V. Barrington

No one ever said that being an internal evaluator was easy. It's Friday night and you're driving home in a downpour, mulling over your less-than-satisfactory meeting with the superintendent. It's hard to see through the windshield past the driving rain, and your mind is not on the road. You need to figure out what to do next.

"Do I go hard core," you wonder, "and really press the methodological issues? Do I cave in and give up my hard-earned credibility with the school system? Is there a middle ground that I can't see clearly yet?"

You walk into the darkened house and begin to pace. Your husband is out of town working on a mediation project, and you have the place to yourself. In the kitchen, you flip on the light switch and pour yourself a glass of wine. You decide to spend the evening working through this quandary: "Why not use my evaluation skills on myself? I'll start by describing the problem." You grab a pen and paper and sit down at the kitchen table.

THE STAKEHOLDERS

The Internal Evaluator

You are the internal evaluator in a large school district and have the lofty title of director of program evaluation. How proud you were when you were hired for this job 3 years ago! Of course, there are distinct challenges to this role. Compared with your external evaluator colleagues, you may be seen as less objective (Love, 2005), be perceived to have more to gain or lose from evaluation findings, and are more likely to experience a conflict of interest (Barrington, 2005). On the other hand, there are some clear advantages to the internal role. You have better relationships with staff, know more about your school system's programs, context, and political processes, and have a greater chance of feeding crucial information into the system's planning cycle in a timely fashion (Love, 2005). You report directly to the new superintendent, and many in the school system are envious of your position.

However, you need to work on your profile within the organization because, during these first 3 years, you have focused on school accreditation, a pet project of the former superintendent. You've had few opportunities to evaluate specific programs, but the work that you have accomplished has provided you with valuable insights into the many records, databases, and networks currently being used in the system.

You know that you can do a good job with this peer-mentoring program evaluation. In your view, the current tools are very weak. You can just imagine what your PhD supervisor/mentor would say if he saw them. "Customer satisfaction surveys!" he would hiss. "A waste of time!" However, you don't want to develop the reputation of being an ivory tower academic. The superintendent's words are still ringing in your ears, and his attitude is pretty clear.

The Superintendent

The superintendent is new to his job, coming from a smaller school district where he developed a strong reputation for having a student-centered focus. He supports the concept of peer mentoring and likes working with that particular age group. You have seen him in action in the schools and know that the kids love him, and as a result so do the teachers. He is an advocate of evaluation and needs to bring some successful evaluation results to the board not only to justify his expenditure of funds but also to garner their support for similar projects (and evaluations) in the future.

He wants to develop a good relationship with the CSA. It is a prestigious agency, and he no doubt heard about them in his former job. Now he has a chance to work with CSA directly. Having freed up funds to evaluate peer mentoring, he may be thinking about additional initiatives. Perhaps he wants CSA to ask him to copresent a paper about peer mentoring at a national research conference next spring. Maybe he would like to serve on a statewide committee on peer mentoring. There are lots of opportunities that a successful superintendent with a positive evaluation report can explore. There aren't enough positive evaluations around!

The Community Services Agency

The CSA has an excellent reputation in the city for its development and implementation of prevention-oriented programs for youth. This group of educational psychologists, social workers, curriculum developers, and youth workers is both dynamic and ambitious. Their peer-mentoring program is being adopted around the state. CSA is happy that your school system has joined their group of clients, and they plan to target even more school districts in the future. Each district that adopts the program pays both an initiation fee for staff training and a per-capita user fee for materials.

Of course, as an evaluator, you have strong opinions about their limited knowledge of evaluation and evaluation processes. In particular, their view on measuring impacts seems to be formulaic and lacking in systems thinking. As an evaluator, you can see the gap between program outcomes and what is being measured, but this is obviously not clear to them. Further, they are using the results from the satisfaction measures as testimonials in their promotional materials; this suggests a fairly strong investment in maintaining the status quo without thinking about it too deeply.

Suddenly, you look up from your notes. This analysis is working. You feel less upset now; maybe there really is a solution. You have a clearer idea of the current situation, but where do you go from here?

THE GUIDING PRINCIPLES FOR EVALUATORS

You rummage through your mail for a brochure you recently received from the American Evaluation Association summarizing the Guiding Principles for Evaluators (American Evaluation Association, 2004). At first glance they all seem to apply to this situation:

1. Systematic Inquiry: You are trying to promote it.
2. Competence: You are attempting to demonstrate it as an internal evaluator.
3. Integrity/Honesty: You have displayed it by voicing your concerns about the current tools.
4. Respect for People: You are endeavoring to ensure it so that participants get the most out of the peer-mentoring program.
5. Responsibilities for General and Public Welfare: You are making an effort to understand these responsibilities in terms of the diversity of stakeholder interests and values in this evaluation.

This last Guiding Principle strikes a chord, and you read it more closely:

Evaluators articulate and take into account the diversity of general and public interests and values . . . [and] should include relevant perspectives and interests of the full range of stakeholders . . . [and] consider not only immediate operations and outcomes of whatever is being evaluated, but also its broad assumptions, implications and potential side effects. (American Evaluation Association, 2004, Principles E, E-1, E-2)

"That's it!" you exclaim. "This is an issue of differing interests. We all want something different and that's why we can't agree."

You take a fresh sheet of paper and begin to brainstorm a list of stakeholder interests. The following table emerges (see Table 3.1).

You stare at what you have just constructed. It's raining so heavily now that there's a wall of sound around the house. It drowns out all thoughts except those focused on your immediate problem. Where are the commonalities of interest? "It's obvious," you conclude. "We want to serve kids and we don't want to fight. That's encouraging, but I need a strategy for what to do next."

TABLE 3.1. Stakeholders' Interests in the Damp Parade Case

Evaluator's interests	Superintendent's interests	CSA's interests
Keep my job	Garner board support	Earn fees through peer-mentoring program expansion
Be a competent evaluator	Support evaluation activities	Minimize change to current evaluation tools
Be methodologically sound	Get approval/funding for additional projects	Use current brochures for marketing purposes
Develop a good working relationship with the superintendent	Develop a good relationship with CSA	Develop a good relationship with your school district
Gain credibility in the school system	Be innovative; gain community support	Look good in the community
Serve kids through collecting appropriate data for decision makers	Serve kids through sound programming	Serve kids through providing sound psychological services and programs
Avoid conflict	Avoid conflict	Avoid conflict

GETTING TO YES

You spot your husband's well-thumbed copy of the Harvard Negotiation Project's *Getting to Yes: Negotiating Agreement without Giving in* (Fisher & Ury, 1991) on the coffee table in the living room. He had been refreshing his memory in preparation for a community project he is working on this weekend in a neighboring state. The book is open to a chapter entitled "Inventing Options for Mutual Gain." As you settle down onto the sofa to read, you're thinking, "I'm going to like this."

> As valuable as it is to have many options, people involved in a negotiation rarely sense a need for them. In a dispute, people usually believe that they know the right answer—their view should prevail.... All available answers appear to lie along a straight line between their position and yours. (Fisher & Ury, 1991, p. 57)

Fisher and Ury see four major obstacles inhibiting the creation of options. You mull over each one in turn.

Judging Prematurely

Premature judgment is certainly true in this case. It is reflected in language imbued with emotion that underscores a judgment or possible bias. The CSA folks call your suggestion "methodological overkill"; the superintendent implies that you seek a "bullet-proof, gold-standard, methodologically pristine type of study." If colored language is an indicator of premature judgment, it sounds like the superintendent has even more of an investment in his perspective than the CSA group has in theirs. Of course, you are not without your own biases as well. You remember your imagined discussion with your former supervisor about customer satisfaction surveys. Hissing could certainly be construed as an emotional response.

Searching for the Single Answer

It is true that your answer (*Change the tools*) is different from their answer (*Leave the tools alone*). Escalation toward a conflict is emerging from the perceived need for one of those answers to be the "winner."

Assuming That the Options Are Dichotomous

Fisher and Ury call this assuming that the pie is a fixed size (Fisher & Ury, 1991, p. 59). This means that the issue is seen in either/or terms. Why bother trying to invent more options if all of them are obvious? It's already a zero-sum game, so there is bound to be a winner and a loser.

"We started out collaborating. Where did it break down?" Then you remember. The early meetings with the CSA team went well, and you were able to achieve consensus on the study design. It was when you started to discuss specific measurement tools that disagreement surfaced. It suddenly became *our tools* versus *your tools*. No other possibilities were considered.

Thinking That "Solving Their Problem Is Their Problem"

This involves each party trying to address its immediate interests. Emotional investment in a particular side of an issue makes it difficult to consider the interests of the other party. As Fisher and Ury (1991) comment, "Shortsighted self-concern thus leads [the parties] . . . to develop only partisan positions, partisan arguments, and one-sided solutions" (p. 59). Although the superintendent says that he is leaving the issue up to you, his implicit message is "I want to look good at the board meeting—Don't rock the boat."

LOOKING FOR OPTIONS FOR MUTUAL GAIN

Fortunately, there is a way out (Fisher & Ury, 1991, p. 60). After reading over Fisher and Ury's suggestions, you arrive at a four-step process to generate possibilities for shared gain:

1. Withhold judgment.
2. Broaden your options.
3. Search for mutual gains.
4. Make their decision easy.

Withhold Judgment

You need to withhold judgment, just as one does in a brainstorming exercise. That seems easier now than it was a few hours ago. It is obvious that your need to be a good evaluator (which also means using sound evaluation methods) is not a need that the other stakeholders necessarily share. It is your professional imperative, not theirs. But maybe your profession can provide more alternatives than you originally thought, which leads to the second step.

Broaden Your Options

What could you do *in conjunction with* the current tools to determine whether the peer-mentoring program is successful? Perhaps a more qualitative approach would produce useful findings that haven't been considered yet. For example, case studies might be employed to explore the implementation process in a few schools. Stake (1995, p. 16) suggests that a case study that is structured around a particular issue can focus attention on complexity and contextuality. What is it about the way the program is offered that makes it more or less successful? Undoubtedly, much goes on in the peer-mentoring program at the individual-school level that can't be captured by a standardized instrument. The wheels in your evaluator's brain begin to turn.

A related option would be to take the most successful schools and find out why they are succeeding; you could work with staff to identify some best practices. You know that evidence-based practice is a growing trend in health care settings (Pape, 2003). You also know that Patton (2001, p. 331) prefers the terms "better" or "effective" practices because the context in which they occur has a critical effect on outcome. Even termed more modestly as "lessons learned," the concept has merit, representing principles extrapolated from multiple sources and triangulated to increase transferability in the form of cumulative knowledge (Patton, 2001, p. 334). It would be particularly helpful for new schools coming into the program to be able to gain from practitioner knowledge that had been validated in some rigorous way.

Or you could use the success case method (Brinkerhoff, 2003) to find out quickly what is working and what is not. On the basis of school means for specific items on the current instruments, you could randomly select, from a subset of high- and/or low-performing schools, several schools for further study. Then you could interview program coordinators, other staff, and even students involved in peer mentoring to better understand which parts of the program are working and which are not.

In 10 minutes, you have come up with three evaluation options that no one had considered. What was the fuss all about?

Search for Mutual Gains

It is important to develop a sense of which options will be the most beneficial for the most players. Another table is forming in your mind and you jot it down (see Table 3.2). It looks like case studies may be less attractive than either the best practices analysis or the success case interviews. However, if you are learning anything from this process, it is that stakeholders' interests may not be readily apparent. It is not a good idea to assume what their interests are. Rather than taking a stand yourself (and defending it at all costs), it makes more sense to present the options to the group, provide the necessary background information, and allow them to consider the pros and cons of each.

Still hovering in the back of your mind is the potential value of organizational records. Your experience with school accreditation has taught you that a great deal of data is readily available in school districts but yet is seldom used. There is bound to be some useful information available that can shed light on the impact of peer mentoring: attendance records, incident reports, standardized test scores, and the like.

Make Their Decision Easy

Because getting what you want depends on the other stakeholders making a decision you can live with, you want to facilitate that pro-

TABLE 3.2. Options for Mutual Gain in the Damp Parade Case

Option	Evaluator		Superintendent		CSA	
	Pros	Cons	Pros	Cons	Pros	Cons
Case studies	Develop in-depth understanding of program	Time consuming	Board will like the stories	Opportunity cost—What else could the evaluator be doing?	Could be used as a selling point with other school districts	May provide more information than they desire
Best practices analysis	Opportunity to collaborate with staff	Methodology less familiar	Interesting from pedagogical perspective	Not common in educational circles	Could be used as a selling point with other school districts	Not common in educational circles
Success case interviews	Uses current tools as springboard	Only one representative interviewed per site	Probes program strengths and weaknesses	Not familiar with method	May be perceived intuitively as more valid (use of random selection)	Not familiar with method

cess. In fact, you want them to think that it is the right thing to do. Because all parties agree that it is important to serve kids, a good strategy might be to start there. Then, given that the status quo in terms of measurement seems fine to them (but not to you), you could ease them into a gradual change process by focusing on interesting and beneficial transitional activities (i.e., one of the three qualitative options) that in turn may lead them to the realization that further changes in instrumentation will provide additional, more relevant information.

THE STRATEGY

So what's the plan? You can offer to continue using the current tools for another year while conducting additional qualitative research activities to "flesh out" the information they are currently obtaining. The stakeholders can select their preferred method from your set of options. In addition, you will also be conducting an analysis of some key school records, selected by you based on your knowledge of the system.

By postponing for a year the tough decision about which new standardized instruments to use and by conducting additional qualitative research in the interim, everyone's understanding of peer-mentoring programs will be enriched. There will be more information available to inform future decisions about ongoing measurement. Who knows what other methodological innovations the stakeholders may be ready to consider at that point?

As Fisher and Ury note, if you make the pie bigger (i.e., generate more options), you move away from a win–lose situation and develop more room within which to negotiate. In your case, you are also "sweetening the pot" by offering more data (Fisher & Ury, 1991, p. 70).

Suddenly, it's quiet. You rise from the sofa and stretch. It's been a long night. The rain has stopped, and you open the front door. You can smell the spruce trees across the street, and you take a deep breath, feeling a lot better now. In fact, you are looking forward to the Monday morning meeting with CSA at which you will present some exciting new options to find out more about peer mentoring.

You aren't going to rain on their parade; in fact, you hope that all of you will soon be celebrating the rich evaluation findings that a multimethod approach will generate. The kids will benefit because the program will improve. The superintendent will be happy because the

Board of Education will be impressed by the evaluation results and the story it tells. The CSA professionals will be pleased because they will learn at least one new research method. They will also have a year to use up their old brochures! Most of all, you will be happy, not only because you will be seen as flexible, easy to work with, and innovative but because you will have done the right thing on ethical grounds by addressing the full range of stakeholder interests and the broader implications of your actions as advocated by the principle of Responsibilities for General and Public Welfare.

As you climb into bed, you reflect on the journey you have taken this evening. It feels good to know that you have looked at the problem in an ethical way and that the Guiding Principles have helped you to see through an emotion-fraught situation. You are aware that there is still a risk involved, that the CSA representatives may not embrace your proposal. However, you believe that if you stress the value you place on your good working relationship with them and provide them with some interesting options to consider, they are likely to be receptive.

On the other hand, if your best efforts fail and everyone remains wedded to these flawed assessment tools, you have a clearer sense of your own position. Your relationship with the new superintendent is more important to you than winning this particular battle. Of course, over time, if he were to continue to agree with everyone but you, his evaluation advisor, it would probably be wise for you to consider moving on. For now, however, the real benefit is to you. The lesson you have learned today is that, although conflict is bound to happen, having external standards and principles to refer to can clarify your thinking and inform your response. You now have better tools for analysis and greater confidence in your ability as an evaluator to manage difficult situations, ethical and otherwise.

REFERENCES

American Evaluation Association. (2004). *Guiding principles for evaluators* (rev.). Available at *www.eval.org/Publications/GuidingPrinciples.asp*.

Barrington, G. (2005). Independent evaluation. In S. Mathison (Ed.), *Encyclopedia of evaluation* (p. 199). Thousand Oaks, CA: Sage.

Brinkerhoff, R. O. (2003). *The success case method: Find out quickly what's working and what's not*. San Francisco: Berrett-Koehler.

Fisher, R., & Ury, W. (1991). *Getting to yes: Negotiating agreement without giving in* (2nd ed.). New York: Penguin Group.

Love, A. (2005). Internal evaluation. In S. Mathison (Ed.), *Encyclopedia of evaluation* (pp. 206–208). Thousand Oaks, CA: Sage.

Pape, T. M. (2003). Evidence-based nursing practice: To infinity and beyond. *Journal of Continuing Education in Nursing, 34*(4), 154–161.

Patton, M. Q. (2001). Evaluation, knowledge management, best practices, and high quality lessons learned. *American Journal of Evaluation, 22*, 329–336.

Stake, R. E. (1995). *The art of case study research.* Thousand Oaks, CA: Sage.

■   ■   ■   ■

WHAT IF . . . ?

. . . the peer-mentoring program has been in place for 5 years rather than just 1?

. . . the superintendent explicitly backs away from his initial request for an impact evaluation, saying that his information needs will be met by a straightforward satisfaction survey?

. . . the superintendent recommends that representatives from the Board of Education be invited to participate in the discussion of outcome measures?

FINAL THOUGHTS

The Damp Parade?

"There must be something in the water."

This saying is apparently more than just a cliché because how else can we explain the independent decisions of our two commentators to take the scenario's title as a point of departure for constructing rain-themed discussions? Although their streams of analysis follow different paths, they end up flowing into adjacent ponds of recommendations.

Mark enters this case through the port of methodology, specifically the Guiding Principle of Systematic Inquiry. He questions whether the type of evaluation being considered for the peer-mentoring program—an impact study with at least some summative overtones—is an appropriate one given the maturity of the program, the possible availability of meta-analyses, and other contextual factors. Indeed, he even questions the wisdom of using organizational record data that the evaluator sees as potentially valuable. For Mark, a successful working through of these issues might reveal that the ethical conflicts facing the evaluator are not nearly as serious as they first seem. And the conflicts that remain, involving the Integrity/Honesty principle and the threat of misuse, are likely to be quite manageable.

Barrington, on the other hand, does not contest, at least initially, the evaluator's depiction of the methodological dimensions of the study. Rather, she focuses on the interests of three major stakeholders in the case (evaluator, CSA, and superintendent), framing her analysis in terms of the principle of Responsibilities for General and Public Welfare. For Barrington, the evaluator's major ethical challenge is to be responsive to multiple stakeholders in designing the study. Although this goal is shared by Mark, he does not accept the evaluator's description of design issues as a coherent, compelling one. Thus, the first order of business for him is dealing with Systematic Inquiry issues.

In the end, both Barrington and Mark recommend that the evaluator take a step back and rethink the design of the study, perhaps opting for a less demanding methodology *now* as a way of establishing a foundation for a more rigorous evaluation *later*. Barrington emphasizes the qualitative–quantitative dimension in discussing this shift, while Mark focuses on formative–summative concerns. In addition, Barrington sees the CSA as the primary target of the evaluator's response, whereas Mark's attention is directed more toward the superintendent.

The ethical importance of generating a shared vision that links an evaluation's purpose with its design is underscored by our commentators' analyses. In the scenario, the superintendent's request for an impact evaluation represents just the starting point for developing such a vision. Much more dialogue needs to occur before a fully formed plan can emerge. Otherwise, the evaluation runs the risk of satisfying neither the requirements of sound social research nor the needs of key stakeholders. Addressing this challenge at the beginning of a project is a core responsibility for evaluators who want to avoid raining on their stakeholders' parades.

What's under the Rock?

New Directions, a private, not-for-profit agency that offers after-school programs for troubled youth, significantly expanded its services 2 years ago to include a tutoring component staffed by adult volunteers. You are an external evaluator who has been hired by New Directions to conduct an outcome evaluation of the tutoring program. The evaluation has recently been requested, and is being paid for, by a local charitable foundation that has provided major funding for the tutoring initiative.

Initial discussions with the New Directions executive director, the paid staff member who coordinates the tutoring program, and a representative from the foundation have been productive. You are now working on the details of the methodology that will be used in the evaluation, given the study's overall design. However, during this process you have encountered a serious obstacle. The information infrastructure necessary to carry out an adequate evaluation of the tutoring program does not appear to be in place. More specifically, the data that the agency has been gathering about the program and its students are fragmented, disorganized, and incomplete.

This is certainly not what you were anticipating based on your prior conversations with the coordinator of the tutoring program. Immediately following your discovery, you scheduled a meeting with him, when the coordinator offered the following comments:

> "Managing this program has been incredibly challenging. We've attracted many more students and volunteers than we ever thought we would. Keeping track of them has been a nightmare, and record-keeping has never been one of our organization's strengths. We're pretty much a mom-and-pop operation in that respect. We thought that an evaluator would help us improve our management information system, in addition to analyzing the data that we *do* have. We'd rather not have the foundation find out how poorly we've been doing at collecting data, since that could hurt us when we seek grant support in the future—and not just support from this foundation. There's definitely a grapevine out there, and we don't want to get blacklisted."

"Well, this is just terrific," you're thinking to yourself. "First, I was misled, or at least not told the whole truth, about the quality of the data I'd be working with. Second, they'd like me to fix the data-collection system as part of the evaluation, a task that was *not* part of our initial agreement. And the frosting on the cake is that they want to keep this "repair job" under wraps so that the foundation doesn't learn about it."

There seems to be so much wrong with this picture, you hardly know where to begin in responding to it. Even so, you must acknowledge that you have a soft spot in your heart for New Directions. They're a relatively young agency with a small number of highly dedicated staff, none of whom have training in evaluation. It's not surprising that they've gotten themselves into this mess. The question now becomes, to what extent is it your responsibility to help them get out of it? And how could you go about doing so in an ethical fashion?

QUESTIONS TO CONSIDER

1. Have you actually been asked to do anything unethical in this situation?

2. Would you be justified in walking away from this evaluation? Do you have an obligation to renegotiate your contract?

3. If the original grant that New Directions received from the foundation did not require the development of a specific record-keeping system for the tutoring program, does New Directions have a duty to inform the foundation of its problems in this domain? Do you have a duty to inform the foundation of those problems?

4. If you had been hired to conduct a *process* evaluation of the tutoring program, how would this affect the decisions you are now facing?

5. What, if anything, could you have done in your initial discussions with the key stakeholders that might have prevented these problems from occurring?

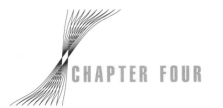

CHAPTER FOUR

Data Collection

The Folder

Nearly a year ago the Safe Neighborhoods Alliance (SNA) was initiated in Dodge, a midwestern city with a population of approximately 130,000. The purpose of SNA is to mobilize residents to work collaboratively to reduce the incidence of violence in Dodge's low-income neighborhoods. SNA is funded by a large private foundation, and SNA's day-to-day operations are overseen by a full-time director who reports to a Governing Board composed of representatives from various constituencies, including parents of school-age children, senior citizens, youth, community activists, and professionals in human services, education, criminal justice, and city government.

You have been hired by the foundation to conduct a process evaluation focusing on SNA's first year of functioning, and for the past several weeks you've been interviewing a wide variety of participants in the alliance. The picture that is emerging from these interviews is one of an organization experiencing growing pains that are typical in community development efforts. In this case, it appears that the director is having difficulty establishing collaborative relationships with a number of key constituencies in the community. The director is in his early 30s and is energetic, optimistic, and very bright. However, his lack of in-depth work experience with community-wide interventions has handicapped his effectiveness thus far.

It is late Tuesday afternoon, and you are waiting for the director to return to his office for the biweekly meeting in which you provide him with an update on the progress of the evaluation. Earlier in the day you had met with Dodge's assistant police chief, who is the chairperson of SNA's Governing Board. He was reviewing crime statistics with you from one of SNA's target neighborhoods when he had to end the meeting abruptly because of an emergency call that required him to go to a crime scene. He apologized profusely and, as he hurried out of the office, handed you a folder labeled "SNA Materials," remarking that "this contains the crime stats we've been talking about, as well as a lot of other info relevant to the evaluation. Feel free to take the folder with you; just make sure to get it back to me before Thursday night's board meeting."

You are perusing the contents of the folder in the director's office when you come across a single page with the heading "Proposal from the Executive Committee." On this page is a draft of a motion to fire the director. A number of justifications for the motion are presented on the sheet. At the bottom of the page, handwritten, are three columns: "Likely in Favor," "Likely Opposed," and "Not Sure." There are a lot of names in the first column and very few in the other two. Thursday's date is written at the top of the page.

You're convinced that the assistant police chief did *not* intend for you to see this document. And you're surprised. You realize that there has been discontent in some quarters with the director's performance, but you did not think that this unhappiness had reached the point at which a termination was being contemplated. Now it looks like the director could be out of a job in the very near future. Personally, you believe that such an action would be premature, given that the Governing Board has not developed a procedure for providing constructive, performance-enhancing feedback to the director.

You wonder whether you are in a position to do *anything* in this situation. For one thing, you're not even supposed to know about what is being proposed. Moreover, what if you do something that results in your being viewed as an ally of the director? Such an outcome could seriously damage the image of professional objectivity that you have worked hard to develop in this evaluation.

As you're mulling over all of this, the director walks briskly into the office. "Sorry I'm late; got held up at a meeting with a subcommittee in the East Side neighborhood. Whew! Dealing with those folks is a real challenge. I've never worked so hard in a job in my life." He flashes you a big grin and laughs. "Hey, you talk with everybody. No one's planning to fire me, are they?"

Hold 'Em or Fold(er) 'Em?: What's an Evaluator to Do?

Michael Hendricks

The Folder scenario could be a poster child for the phrase "Appearances can be deceiving." At first glance, the ethical challenge seems straightforward: How should I respond to the director's question about possibly being fired? Upon further reflection, however, the issues become more involved, the challenge more complex, and the existence of a single "proper" response less obvious. Under certain assumptions, all five of the Guiding Principles for Evaluators (American Evaluation Association, 2004) might reasonably apply, making for a thought-provoking case indeed.

In my opinion, responding to the director's query is a relatively minor issue. Instead, the key ethical issue is whether or not I should become involved in discussions of his future, and that question is what makes this case unusual. In my experience, most ethical challenges relate to *what* evaluators should do in a given situation. For example, I've wrestled with what to do when a client wanted to increase the co-payment for a social service that I felt should actually cost less, what to do when a client wanted me to delete from a report anonymous quotes I thought were necessary, what to do when a client wanted me to remain quiet about information I believed the client needed to hear, and other similar dilemmas. In each case, it was clear that I needed to take some action, but it was not clear what that action should be.

In the present situation, the central ethical question isn't *what* I should do but *whether* I should do anything at all. It is not obvious that the fate of the director is any of my business, so should I become involved? If I do decide to become involved, the question of what to do would then arise, but only then. In my view, the initial, primary ethical question in this case is, "Should I take any action whatsoever in this situation?" As such, I believe this case raises important issues not directly addressed by the Guiding Principles: When is a difficult situation involving an entity being evaluated ethically a part of our evaluation, and when is it ethically separate from the evaluation?

Figure 4.1 illustrates these two possibilities. Circle E represents the SNA evaluation, and the boundary of the circle represents all my activities relevant to the evaluation. This circle encompasses a wide variety of activities, and the size of the circle depends on the scope and complexity of the evaluation and my efforts during the evaluation. That is, a broader or more involved evaluation requires a larger circle than a narrower or less involved evaluation. However, no matter how broad the evaluation or how involved I am, I still have a larger life (Circle L) outside the evaluation, and there are many aspects of my life totally unrelated to my SNA evaluation. My wife, tennis, Spanish lessons, church activities, and a thousand other aspects of my private life clearly fall within Circle L but outside Circle E.

As a result of having a private life, each day I face ethical challenges outside Circle E but inside Circle L. If I find a cash-filled wallet on the street, I certainly face an ethical challenge, but this challenge has nothing to do with my ongoing evaluations. As I ponder what to do with the wallet, the Guiding Principles may offer general guidance for Integrity/Honesty or Respect for People, but in their essence the Guiding Principles are fundamentally irrelevant to what I do with the wallet. This is a significant point highlighted by this case, and it raises interesting issues that the next revision of the Guiding Principles might address.

However, what if the cash-filled wallet begins to filter into the case at hand? What if the wallet belongs to the assistant police chief, who is also the chair of the Governing Board? Furthermore, what if I find the wallet in the parking lot immediately after meeting with the chair on my way to meet with the director? Do these highly personalizing facts bring the ethical challenge within the scope of my SNA evaluation, that is, within Circle E?

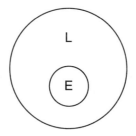

FIGURE 4.1. Relationship between life experience (L) and SNA evaluation experience (E).

Not at all, at least in my opinion. Nothing about the situation has changed except the unfortunate loser of the wallet, and so the situation still falls outside the ethical boundaries of the SNA evaluation. Obviously other ethical guidelines do apply, based on my culture, religious beliefs, humanistic tendencies, and basic morality, and I am personally quite clear as to what I would do. However, even though the wallet now belongs to an evaluation-related individual and is found during evaluation-related activities, neither of these facts justifies invoking a special set of principles that are explicitly "intended to guide the professional practice of evaluators" (American Evaluation Association, 2004, Preface-C).

Keeping in mind the distinction between those ethical challenges that fit inside my professional practice and those that fall outside it, let us consider the case situation as presented, from both a more conservative and a more liberal perspective, not in the political meanings of those words but in the purer sense of making fewer or more assumptions. From a conservative perspective, and focusing simply on the available facts, the situation seems clear: Accidentally reading about the director's possible firing is ethically identical to finding the chair's wallet in the parking lot. Both situations are unfortunate for the person involved, but neither situation invokes the Guiding Principles, because neither situation falls within Circle E. That is, neither situation compels me to act in my role *as evaluator* of the SNA program.

Moreover, and more strongly, neither situation even *allows* me to act. I believe the Guiding Principles offer at least four possible prohibitions from becoming involved in the situation:

1. Commenting on the director's job performance is not a part of my evaluation assignment. The Integrity/Honesty principle urges me to "negotiate honestly with clients and relevant stakeholders concerning the . . . tasks to be undertaken" (American Evaluation Association, 2004, Principle C-1), and I've been hired specifically "to conduct a process evaluation focusing on SNA's first year of functioning." My assignment makes no mention of evaluating personnel or their performance, and to do so would violate my contract with the foundation.

2. Even if the board were to solicit my opinion of the director's performance despite that issue being outside my assignment, I have no systematic information to offer. The Systematic Inquiry principle encourages me to "make clear the limitations of [my] evaluation and its results" (American Evaluation Association, 2004, Principle A-3), and the Integrity/Honesty principle indicates that I should "not

misrepresent [my] procedures, data or findings" (Principle C-5). In reality, I've been collecting data for only "the past several weeks," a very brief period of time, certainly not long enough to have developed "a comprehensive understanding of the important contextual elements of the evaluation" (Principle D-1), as the Respect for People principle recommends.

3. Nothing about my evaluation can be construed to have triggered the possible firing of the director. That is, there is no indication that either the processes I have engaged in (interviews conducted, meetings held, or issues raised that would not have occurred without the evaluation) or the results from the evaluation (preliminary findings of any sort) have contributed to the memo. If it were otherwise (i.e., if an aspect of my evaluation could be linked with the firing possibility) then a number of Guiding Principles would become relevant, including Respect for People, which encourages me to act in order to "maximize the benefits and reduce any unnecessary harms that might occur" (American Evaluation Association, 2004, Principle D-3). However, my evaluation is not responsible for the topic arising.

4. The Respect for People principle also urges me to "conduct the evaluation and communicate its results in a way that clearly respects the stakeholders' dignity and self worth" (American Evaluation Association, 2004, Principle D-4), and the Responsibilities for General and Public Welfare principle states that I should "include relevant perspectives and interests of the full range of stakeholders" (Principle E-1). The director is clearly an important stakeholder in this evaluation, but so is the board. If I presume that my limited information gained over several weeks is more relevant for a crucial personnel decision than the board's collective knowledge gained by working with the director for "nearly a year," am I respecting these stakeholders, especially if I have not interviewed the board about their perspectives on the director? It is important to remember that the board includes "representatives from various constituencies," some of whom are "professionals in human services, education, criminal justice, and city government." These experienced persons have hired and fired before, they will do it again, and they deserve my respect.

From this conservative perspective, then, the proper action is no action at all. The director's fate is appropriately an issue for others, and I should remain uninvolved. On a practical level, I would mirror the director's laughing question by responding with a lighthearted "Well, if they were, I doubt they'd be confiding in me" and then proceed with the meeting as I would normally. This response is not only true (in fact, no one did confide in me about this issue), but it also deflects the director's anxiety and quickly moves on. I would return the file to the chair as soon as possible, explain that I am sure he never intended for me to read the memo, assure him I haven't talked with anyone about it, and promise not to do so in the future. Oh, yes, one more thing: Unless there is a good reason not to, I would definitely attend Thursday's board meeting to see what happens.

If this is the conservative perspective, what might be a more liberal one? In this instance, I contrast the words *liberal* and *conservative* to suggest that, although a conservative might consider only the facts at hand, a liberal might entertain the possibility that there are *implications* of the situation that are important to take into account. Could a more liberal perspective draw different conclusions about the proper actions to take?

In particular, the case mentions that I have already come to realize that the SNA is "an organization experiencing growing pains that are typical in community development efforts." But how do I know that these growing pains are typical? Apparently, this isn't my first time evaluating this sort of program; if I describe growing pains as "typical," it is likely that I have had relevant prior experience. If so, does my experience with similar programs change the ethical calculations? Is it now ethically *permitted*, or perhaps even ethically *required*, for me to offer my experience to this discussion?

I believe the answer depends on the extent and type of my experience, and Figure 4.2 clarifies the different possibilities. Circles E and L remain the same, representing my SNA evaluation (E) and my larger life (L) outside the evaluation. But these two Euler circles are now joined by Circle PE, representing my prior evaluation experience. By definition, all experienced evaluators possess a storehouse of knowledge based on their previous evaluation work, and quite often something in this storehouse is relevant when we begin a new evaluation. Might Circle PE require me to rethink my conservative decision not to become involved?

I would argue that the answer depends on the specific relationship between Circle E and Circle PE. Figure 4.2a, for example, reflects a scenario in which I have evaluation experience, perhaps even considerable experience, but none of it is relevant to the current evaluation. Perhaps my experience has been with completely different types of

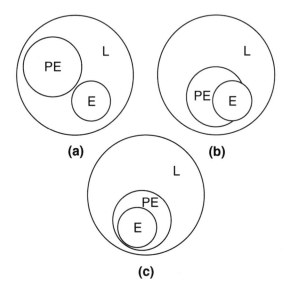

FIGURE 4.2. Possible relationships between life experience (L), previous evaluation experience (PE), and SNA evaluation experience (E).

programs, perhaps the programs were similar but the contexts quite different, or perhaps the programs and contexts were similar but I didn't evaluate director–community relations. In any event, Figure 4.2a is ethically identical to Figure 4.1, and neither scenario justifies my becoming involved in the discussion about firing the director. It is not my business, and I have nothing to add.

Figures 4.2b and 4.2c, however, reflect a different type of experience, and the difference is noteworthy. They offer the possibility that, ethically, perhaps I should become involved. Figure 4.2b shows that some (but not all) of the current evaluation falls within my prior evaluation experience. That is, I'm not intimately familiar with all aspects of the current evaluation (the nonoverlapping parts of Circles E and PE), but I've also evaluated similar programs in the past (the overlapping part of the two circles). In this scenario, my experience evaluating a director's relationship with the community becomes a critical factor in deciding whether I should act.

Similarly, but even more persuasively, Figure 4.2c shows that *all* of the current SNA evaluation falls within my prior experience. That is, everything about this evaluation is familiar to me. Perhaps I am a highly respected expert on exactly this type of community develop-ment alliance, with many years of working with dozens of similar alli-ances and the public recognition to prove it. In fact, the foundation may have specifically recruited me for this evaluation because of my reputation for excellence in these process evaluations.

In either of these two scenarios, where the current evaluation overlaps either partially (Figure 4.2b) or completely (Figure 4.2c) with my evaluation experience, several Guiding Principles suggest that it might be reasonable to involve myself in the discussion about firing the director.

- The Competence principle indicates that I should "possess (or ensure that the evaluation team possesses) the education, abilities, skills, and experience appropriate to undertake the tasks proposed in the evaluation" (American Evaluation Association, 2004, Principle B-1). Although I have not yet systematically studied the issue of director–community relations in the current evaluation, my experience has taught me how these relations typically develop elsewhere. This expe-rience gives me relevant insights not known to anyone else in Dodge.

- The Integrity/Honesty principle states that if I "determine that certain procedures or actions are likely to produce misleading eval-uative information or conclusions, [I] have the responsibility to com-municate [my] concerns and the reasons for them" (American Evalua-tion Association, 2004, Principle C-6). Although the procedures and actions in this instance are board based and not evaluation based, my experience tells me that the board may be taking a serious step based on information and conclusions that I believe are misleading. If so, I seem to have a responsibility to communicate my concerns.

- The Respect for People principle urges me to "seek a compre-hensive understanding of the important contextual elements of the evaluation" (American Evaluation Association, 2004, Principle D-1). Previous evaluations have taught me that it is typical for director–community relations to have growing pains, yet the board appears not to realize this. Therefore, I am in a unique position to put the "discon-tent in some quarters with the director's performance" into a proper context over the life of a program.

- The Respect for People principle also encourages me to "maxi-mize the benefits and reduce any unnecessary harms that might occur" during the evaluation (American Evaluation Association, 2004, Princi-ple D-3). Again, even though the harm to the program would not result from any aspect of my evaluation, my background gives me a unique ability to help the Board avoid taking a precipitous or dangerous action.

• Finally, the Responsibilities for General and Public Welfare principle asserts that I should "consider not only the immediate operations and outcomes of whatever is being evaluated, but also its broad assumptions, implications and potential side effects" (American Evaluation Association, 2004, Principle E-2). In this instance, the board is negatively evaluating the director's performance, and I believe that their assumptions are incorrect and that their too-hasty actions may produce harmful implications and side effects for the program.

None of these five arguments provides, in my view, total justification for becoming involved. Each Guiding Principle addresses how I should conduct the evaluation, not how the Board should conduct its discussion of the director's fate. However, the spirit of the Guiding Principles is certainly that information should be presented, and decisions taken, with a full understanding of the facts and the total context. In that regard, the principles open the door to my possible involvement, but they certainly do not require it. An ethical decision would still remain.

However, if I do decide to become involved, I would then find myself in a more typical ethical scenario, as discussed at the beginning of this commentary, that is, determining what to do. In this instance, more than 48 hours remain before the board meeting, so I have sufficient time to act carefully. And carefully is exactly how I should act, because I might be reading too much into what I have read, another example of "appearances may be deceiving." For example, I believe the following uncertainties are very relevant:

• The memo is only a draft of a proposed motion, not a final motion itself.

• Who drafted the memo? The Executive Committee? The chair? A member of the Executive Committee? Is it even a genuine motion, or possibly only a planted attempt to use me to stir unrest by raising the issue with the director or others?

• The three columns of names may indicate only how the chair assumes different board members will feel about the proposal, not necessarily the results of an actual polling of their views.

• Thursday's date written on the proposal may signify only that the chair plans to begin discussing it with board members at that meeting, not that the motion will actually be introduced and officially deliberated upon.

- The justifications listed in the proposal may simply be an acceptable public cover for the actual reasons for firing the director. In reality, perhaps the director is in trouble over transgressions the board prefers to keep private, such as financial misconduct, unwanted sexual advances, or a distortion of the director's credentials. If so, my evaluation experience may be relevant to the public issues but not to the actual issues.

- The chair may, for whatever reasons, decide to shelve the idea before Thursday's meeting.

These six uncertainties create valid reasons to proceed with caution, and any one of the six might make me reconsider whether to become involved at all. However, the case description suggests one other reason for caution, which, in my opinion, is *not* an ethically valid reason. In the case description, I worry "what if [I] do something that results in [me] being viewed as an ally of the director? Such an outcome could seriously damage the image of professional objectivity that [I] have worked hard to develop in this evaluation." I certainly understand the practical concerns involved, and I would certainly not want to mar my reputation with any of the stakeholders, but I believe the Guiding Principles allow me no latitude to withhold important information simply because sharing it might make my job more difficult. In fact, several Guiding Principles clearly urge me to share all relevant information without consideration of how it affects me personally. That is, however I decide to act, I should not weigh too heavily the ramifications for me professionally.

If, therefore, it still seems appropriate to become involved, I would approach the chair privately that same day, return the file, explain what I've read, and ask to discuss the issue. I would then inquire if the director's job is, in fact, under discussion. If so, I would explain my prior experience, what I've learned across other settings about the development of director–community relations, and why I believe it may be premature to fire the director.

I would listen to the chair's reactions, and if he agrees that my experience is relevant, I would ask his advice on how to introduce my experience into the discussion. If the chair agrees that I should become involved, I would advise him that I need to talk immediately with my client at the foundation, since the Responsibilities for General and Public Welfare principle acknowledges that "[e]valuators necessarily have a special relationship with the client who funds or requests the evalua-tion" (American Evaluation Association, 2004, Principle E-4). I would then discuss the entire situation with the foundation and "record all changes made in the originally negotiated project plans, and the rea-sons why the changes were made" (Principle C-3).

If, however, the chair does *not* believe that my experience is rele-vant to the situation and is *not* willing to involve me in the discussions, my options become more complicated. To press the issue further would almost certainly irritate and possibly alienate the chair, causing difficulties throughout the remainder of the evaluation. On the other hand, I may believe it is important to raise the issue with my founda-tion client, given my concern about the potential harm to the program. At this point, deciding whether to continue becomes a situation-specific calculation of the trade-offs between the potential risks versus the potential benefits, and it is impossible to offer general guidance.

Throughout these conversations, and regardless of how they con-clude, it is ethically important that I make others aware, and remain acutely aware myself, of the personal values motivating my urge to become involved. According to the Integrity/Honesty principle, I should "be explicit about [my] own . . . interests and values concerning the conduct and outcomes of an evaluation" (American Evaluation Association, 2004, Principle C-4). My interest in the case is not value free; I care about the director's fate because "personally, [I] believe that such an action would be premature, given that the Governing Board has not developed a procedure for providing constructive, performance-enhancing feedback to the director."

Although these concerns may seem quite appropriate to me, they spring from personal values I bring to the situation: that firing some-one is a radical step, that it should be avoided if possible, that a board has certain obligations to a director, that one of those obligations is to provide feedback to the director, that part of that feedback should help enhance the director's performance, that a director should not be fired until given a chance to improve performance, and so on. Other persons may share these values, or they may not. Before acting, I need to recog-nize that I act at least partly *because* of these values, not because I have systematic, objective evaluation information to offer.

I believe these are the ethical issues inherent in this case, and this is my analysis of them from both a more conservative and a more lib-eral perspective. But might the ethics have been different under a somewhat different set of circumstances? In particular, are there conditions under which another set of actions would have been more appropriate? I see two main possibilities.

First, if my contract with the foundation had clearly required from the beginning a personnel evaluation of the director's performance, then I almost certainly would have established criteria of successful performance, gathered information from a wide variety of sources, analyzed and interpreted that information in the most transparent manner possible, shared both preliminary and final conclusions with all stakeholders, and jointly developed recommendations for next steps. It seems highly unlikely that the board would consider firing the director until this process ran its course, and if they did, I would have solid ethical grounds to object (see C-1 of the Integrity/Honesty principle).

The second possibility involves the fact that, after only a few weeks, I already "realize[d] that there has been discontent in some quarters with the director's performance." Had I appreciated the full extent of this discontent, I could have discreetly raised the issue with my foundation client and possibly renegotiated my contract (see C-3 of the Integrity/Honesty principle) to include an explicit examination of the director's performance. Alternatively, had I shared my initial concerns with the foundation at this early stage, it might have suggested the renegotiation. In either event, the result would almost certainly have been to forestall board action as noted previously.

In conclusion, the "proper" ethical action to take in The Folder case can be summarized as, "It depends." I realize this is not necessarily the most prescriptive advice, but prescriptive advice may not be common in ethical discussions. In my view, ethics is a process, not an outcome: it is the process of continually questioning our actions in every situation. In this instance, assumptions we make about the relevance of our prior evaluation experience seem to determine the range of ethically acceptable options.

REFERENCE

American Evaluation Association. (2004). *Guiding principles for evaluators* (rev.). Available at *www.eval.org/Publications/GuidingPrinciples.asp*.

COMMENTARY

Centering the Folder

sarita davis

The role of the evaluator has been debated for decades. There are multiple and layered positions, ranging from advocate to adversary and partisan to nonpartisan (Datta, 1999). I suspect where one falls on this continuum is largely influenced by his or her geopolitical worldview. I am an African American woman committed to liberation and self-determination for oppressed communities, especially those of African descent. My favored evaluation frameworks emphasize co-construction (Thomas, 2004), collaboration (Greene, 1988; Patton, 1997), cultural competence (Frierson, Hood, & Hughes, 2002), empowerment (Fetterman, 2000), feminism (Stanley & Wise, 1983), inclusiveness (Mertens, 1999), multiculturalism (Kirkhart, 1995), stakeholder participation (Cousins & Earl, 1995), and responsiveness (House, 2001; Stake, 1975). These approaches represent the best of our evaluation knowledge with regard to engaging stakeholders, identifying multiple meanings, partnering with participants, valuing culture/customs/norms, and exploring context. Ultimately, they all endeavor to bring us closer to understanding the evaluation question of the moment.

Given this background, it should not be surprising that I strongly lean toward the roles of evaluator as partisan and advocate. Consequently, it is from this position that I frame my approach to The Folder scenario. The goal of my response is to highlight opportunities that expand inclusion, increase dialogue, and support deliberation. I will do this from a perspective that attempts to "center" the commentary in the particular history and culture of the community in which the evaluation is taking place.

CENTERING

I would argue that the issues raised in The Folder scenario (e.g., disclosure, accountability, and allegiance) must be considered within the context of larger, truth-seeking concerns such as commitment to fairness and the public good. Of course, neither the Guiding Principles for Evaluators nor any other set of professional guidelines can guarantee the practice of its tenets. One reason is that socially learned biases that can affect our behavior are systemically woven into the fabric of society; consider the strong public response to *Crash*, the 2005 Academy Award-winning film that focused on the multiple "isms" that lay just below the surface of so many of our interactions. Americans tend to uphold "perspectivelessness" theories that minimize the importance of race, class, and gender. This stance is problematic because it encourages race-conscious individuals to adopt a worldview fostering White middle-class values that claim to carry no such orientation (Crenshaw, 1989). One result is that those who are sensitive to the pervasiveness of race, class, and gender bias can seldom ground their analysis in their own experiences without risking some kind of formal or informal sanction. Rather, they are expected to take the position of a distant observer, as if they had no investment or direct contact with the issue.

Marginalized communities, especially communities of color, usually bear the brunt of negative stereotypes. A passive analytical stance that simply calls for opening the floor to "diverse perspectives" does little to mediate the deeply rooted historical issues characterizing these communities. In contrast, a proactive position, such as "centering," defines the evaluation phenomenon from the collective historical, political, and socioeconomic experience of the targeted population.

What is centering? Simply put, it is viewing a phenomenon from the perspective of the targeted community. A basic premise of centering is that culture matters, in the past, the present, and the future. Centering means constructing the inquiry with the history, culture, and geo-political reality of the participants at the very core. For example, in The Folder scenario, if we know the lived experience of the community and begin the evaluation from a centered approach, certain questions arise that would otherwise remain unaddressed. If the community were predominantly African American, its historical and contemporary relationship with law enforcement would become a critical issue, especially since Dodge's assistant police chief is the chairperson of SNA's Governing Board. Distrust and animosity between law enforcement and marginalized communities is a significant centering factor. (Indeed, famed attorney Johnnie Cochran built his career on police misconduct cases reflecting this tension.) On the other hand, if the community's demographics were predominantly European American and blue collar, issues involving policing might be just as volatile but relate primarily to civil liberties and the right to bear arms. Or they might not be volatile at all. Such contextual factors have implications for not only who is involved in the evaluation process, but who is perceived to have power and control.

In the analysis that follows, I will examine The Folder scenario under two sets of centering assumptions, exploring how those assumptions might affect the decisions and actions that the evaluator would deem most ethically appropriate. In Community 1, the target neighborhoods are 80% Caucasian American and 20% Latin American. Most residents are locally employed as manual laborers in blue-collar jobs (e.g., assembly-line workers, construction workers, restaurant servers, secretaries). The neighborhoods are primarily composed of two-parent families, with a median income of $35,000. Quality of life is relatively stable, with most residents remaining in the community from birth to death. It is only recently that crime has become an issue as inner-city residents from other cities have moved into these neighborhoods.

In Community 2, the target neighborhoods are 80% African American and 20% Caribbean immigrants. Employed residents work primarily as front-line workers and midlevel managers in service industry jobs (e.g., auto parts stores, supermarkets, bars, restaurants, health clinics). These neighborhoods have experienced significant growth as a result of an influx of out-of-state residents and immigrants and are mainly composed of two-parent families, with a median income of $25,000.

To inform the analyses that follow, I will incorporate findings from the National Survey of American Life (NSAL). This is a comprehensive and detailed study of racial, ethnic, and cultural influences on mental health in the United States (Jackson et al., 2004). The surveyed adults include blacks of African descent (African Americans), Caribbean descent (Caribbean Blacks), and non-Hispanic Whites (Americans largely of European descent). Supplementary interviews were conducted with African American and Caribbean Black adolescents who were attached to the NSAL adult households. The majority of Caribbean Black youth were from households with family members from Jamaica, Haiti, or Trinidad and Tobago.

The following section has two aims: (1) to identify the ethical challenges raised by the scenario; and (2) to discuss culturally relevant responses of the evaluator depending on the community profile. The conceptual lens of centering that guides this discussion explores the political contexts that influence who constructs the evaluation questions and the resulting decisions. Centering the evaluation challenges evaluators to focus not solely on race/ethnicity, class, gender, nationality, or other forms of difference but also on the intersection of all these factors as both points of cohesion and fracture within groups.

THE ETHICAL CHALLENGES

When viewed from the vantage point of the Guiding Principles, several key ethical issues emerge in this scenario, including transparency, disclosure, and confidentiality. These challenges touch on one or more aspects of each of the Guiding Principles: Systematic Inquiry, Competence, Integrity/Honesty, Respect for People, and Responsibilities for General and Public Welfare. In my judgment, there is one response that is of immediate value to the evaluator in this situation: She should disclose her knowledge of the sensitive information and explain how the impending decision to fire the executive director could negatively impact the evaluation. My other recommendations are methodological strategies that can be used to collect culturally relevant, varied, and comprehensive data that can be used to inform the board's decision to keep or fire the director.

Systematic Inquiry

The Systematic Inquiry principle indicates that "evaluators should explore with the client the shortcomings and strengths both of the various evaluation questions and the various approaches that might be used for answering those questions" (American Evaluation Association, 2004, Principle A-2). In the scenario, the evaluator was hired by the foundation to conduct a process evaluation focusing on SNA's first year of functioning. Because this intervention is in its formative stage, process evaluation is an excellent choice to assess the congruence among what was proposed (program theory), what was presented (program implementation), and what was received (participants' perspectives). The strength of process evaluation is its ability to detect gaps between program theory and practice. However, process findings should not be used as the basis for making summative judgments about this program's impact, especially in its first year of operation.

The Systematic Inquiry principle reinforces the goal of transparency when it recommends that "evaluators should make clear the limitations of an evaluation and its results [and] discuss in a contextually appropriate way those values, assumptions, theories, methods, results, and analyses significantly affecting the interpretation of the evaluative findings" (American Evaluation Association, 2004, Principle A-3). It is evident from the evaluator's unspoken beliefs that a decision to fire the director would be premature, especially since the Governing

Board had not developed a procedure for providing constructive, performance-enhancing feedback to him. Putnam (1990) calls for the use of some type of deliberative process to address such a situation, suggesting that ethical issues are not puzzles to be solved through technical approaches but rather issues to be adjudicated through social deliberation.

What Might Be Done

The events in the scenario clearly have implications for program implementation and the results of the evaluation. An ethical response on the part of the evaluator would encompass raising critical questions about formative versus summative evaluation, the lack of constructive feedback mechanisms, and how this impedes program development and potentially limits the evaluation findings. This overall response would be the same for both community profiles. However, the way in which this feedback would be offered might differ. For example, in Community 1, which has been stable and relatively homogeneous for many years, questions about the potential effects of a premature decision are likely to be taken at face value and perceived as constructive. In contrast, in Community 2, there is a chance that historical influences would cause residents to see this feedback as an attempt to control them and gain power over their decision making.

Although African American and Caribbean families came to America in different ways, their experiences with discrimination appear to be quite similar. For example, respondents from the NSAL survey report experiencing various types of discrimination in their daily lives, such as being treated with less courtesy or as less intelligent than others, being treated poorly by authority figures, or being called names or insulted. Both African American and Caribbean Black males report more types of discrimination than their female counterparts. Discrimination most often was attributed to race or ancestry.

In the case at hand, an ethical response requires that the evaluator address the potential deleterious effects of making changes prematurely. However, given the pervasive feelings of discrimination likely to exist in Community 2, especially among males, this feedback should focus on the *options* emerging from the collective reflection and consideration of the group. In sum, a humble approach of explicitly acknowledging that the final decision is theirs to make is more likely to be heard and accepted.

Competence

Within the context of The Folder scenario, the following passage from the Competence principle is perhaps most relevant: "To ensure recognition, accurate interpretation and respect for diversity, evaluators should ensure that the members of the evaluation team collectively demonstrate cultural competence" (American Evaluation Association, 2004, Principle B-1).

An evaluator can address cultural competence pertaining to the two community profiles in several ways. These include, but are not limited to, observation, interviewing, and review of documentation. In the scenario, interviewing is already being used as a data-collection strategy, so I will focus on the other two methodologies. As indicated earlier, these strategies are offered to help the evaluator obtain diverse and culturally relevant information that will ultimately inform the board's actions concerning the director.

What Might Be Done

Observing the community in which the evaluation takes place is one way to understand community dynamics and the relevant questions to ask and to whom. With roots in natural inquiry, field notes offer context to observations in the form of sight, sound, smell, and touch. Taking such notes is an essential task of the observer in the field; they can provide the evaluator with data for later analysis (Agar, 1980). In The Folder scenario, this journalistic style of reporting can capture the pulse of the community in its diversity and depth of opinions, ultimately offering critical contextual feedback for all stakeholders.

Another approach to developing cultural competence is using existing documentation. A variety of traditional documents and archival materials should be considered, including court records, local community newspapers, electronic/video media, census data, and so forth. These resources would probably be sufficient in Community 1. However, the approaches to discovery in Community 2 will probably require more creativity. Historically, subordinate groups have not had adequate resources or opportunities to air their concerns. Consequently, other types of data—art, for example—can provide the evaluator with valuable information on the lives of individuals in the community, including their history and broad social trends. I might approach local artists, poets, and underground musicians. For example, eating establishments typically display the cultural happenings in a community, especially in Caribbean neighborhoods. By using field notes, archival documentation, and art, the evaluator could increase her cultural competence by contextualizing issues in a way that explores the experience of all constituencies, ascertain the relevant questions to ask, and determine to whom the questions should be addressed. Ultimately, this information would be shared with the funders and other stakeholders so that they are informed by the views and sentiments of the community-at-large before a decision regarding the director is reached.

Integrity/Honesty

According to the Integrity/Honesty principle, "Evaluators should negotiate honestly with clients and relevant stakeholders concerning the costs, tasks to be undertaken, limitations of methodology, scope of results likely to be obtained, and uses of data resulting from a specific evaluation. It is primarily the evaluator's responsibility to initiate discussion and clarification of these matters, not the client's" (American Evaluation Association, 2004, Principle C-1).

In The Folder case, the evaluator comes across a proposal from the Executive Committee to fire the director. This sentiment and potential action have implications that can change the direction, scope, and outcome of the evaluation. The evaluator wonders if she is in a position to do *anything* in this situation. There are obvious conflicts: (1) The evaluator is not supposed to know about the proposal to fire the director; and (2) if she does something, she may be viewed as an ally of the director and ultimately damage the professional image she has tried to develop in the evaluation. In this context, the Guiding Principles clearly compel the evaluator to disclose knowledge of her discovery to *all* stakeholders, first to the funders and then to the other stakeholders associated with the project.

The Integrity/Honesty principle also asserts that "if evaluators determine that certain procedures or activities are likely to produce misleading evaluative information or conclusions, they have the responsibility to communicate their concerns and the reasons for them" (American Evaluation Association, 2004, Principle C-6). Once again, it appears that the evaluator should take a stand and speak to concerns that could negatively impact the evaluation. Some might say that evaluators cannot be fair if they take a position for or against any stakeholder. Regardless of the role assumed by the evaluator, however, the proposed personnel action has implications for the outcome of the evaluation as well as the general and public welfare. Taking an advocacy position in this instance should not be viewed as being for or against a particular group but as supporting a fair hearing of all perspectives (House & Howe, 1998; Ryan, Greene, Lincoln, Mathison, & Mertens, 1998).

What Might Be Done

The ethical response in this situation requires the evaluator to be inclusive of diverse perspectives; it is generally considered the best way to facilitate authentic deliberation (House & Howe, 1998) to resolve conflicting claims (Putnam, 1990). Although there are many methods to accomplish this task of deliberation, concept mapping is especially valuable (Trochim, 1989). It utilizes information from individuals to (1) identify shared understanding within groups; (2) represent group ideas pictorially; (3) encourage teamwork; and (4) facilitate group agreement, decision making, and forward movement. This methodology is rooted in a purposeful use of multiple stakeholders to generate participant-grounded knowledge.

Concept mapping generally assumes that there is an identifiable group responsible for guiding the evaluation or planning effort. In The Folder scenario, this group might consist of the following: community residents and leaders, law enforcement, academicians, policymakers, funding agents, and representatives of community-based organizations, relevant client populations, and other constituencies. The concept mapping process could be overseen by the evaluator, a facilitator, or an internal member of the planning group.

In this scenario, concept mapping is offered as a process for collecting and illustrating varied perspectives for the express purpose of adding breadth and depth to the discussion of the director's performance. This methodology would be ideal for both Community 1 and Community 2. It allows participants to voice issues in their own words and without judgment. The identified concerns can be turned into strategies or action plans that ultimately enhance the evaluation outcome.

Respect for People

There are three aspects of this principle that are especially relevant to The Folder case. The first is that "evaluators should seek a comprehensive understanding of the important contextual elements of the evaluation" (American Evaluation Association, 2004, Principle D-1). The second is that "knowing that evaluations may negatively affect the interests of some stakeholders, evaluators should conduct the evaluation and communicate its results in a way that clearly respects the stakeholders' dignity and self-worth" (Principle D-4). Finally, "evaluators have the responsibility to understand and respect differences among participants . . . and to account for potential implications of these differences when planning, conducting, analyzing, and reporting evaluations" (Principle D-6).

What Might Be Done

Not surprisingly, there is a great deal of overlap between cultural competence and the Respect for People principle. Respect for differences cannot be achieved without listening and actively involving the community (see Smith, 1999). In the context of evaluation, respect is a necessary prerequisite to achieving cultural competence; they are reciprocal. Indeed, the majority of NSAL respondents said that the most frequent type of discrimination they experienced was "people acting as if they were better than them" (Jackson et al., 2004). To act respectfully in The Folder scenario means to actively seek and honor different worldviews among stakeholders and to consider the potential implications of these differences as they relate to the future of the executive director. The evaluator should seek the input of stakeholders in their places of safety, comfort, and choosing: their homes, places of worship, and so forth. Again, a methodology such as concept mapping provides a format for implementing this principle. In the end, the key is to allow stakeholders to tell their stories in their way.

Responsibilities for General and Public Welfare

According to this principle, "Evaluators should consider not only the immediate operations and outcomes of whatever is being evaluated, but also its broad assumptions, implications and potential side effects" (American Evaluation Association, 2004, Principle E-2). When there is a conflict between a client's interests and others' interests, "evaluators should explicitly identify and discuss the conflicts with the client and relevant stakeholders" (Principle E-4). Finally, "clear threats to the public good should never be ignored in any evaluation" (Principle E-5).

In the scenario, the evaluator was hired by a foundation and worked in conjunction with multiple stakeholders on a project that would ultimately benefit low-income neighborhoods. Clearly, there are many constituents with diverse perspectives and political agendas in this situation The Guiding Principles acknowledge that there will be times when the evaluator's work will be at odds with the individuals signing the check. In these circumstances, Guzman and Feria (2002) contend that adaptability in the midst of evaluation is a practical reality and should not be seen as a threat to the validity of the evaluation. In fact, evaluators would be wise to build flexibility into the evaluation timeline. Guzman and Feria maintain that the needs of the stakeholders, the broader community, and the target population are continuously being shaped and adjusted by contextual factors. The ethical response requires the evaluator to advocate for prudence, caution, and a fair hearing of all the information.

What Might Be Done

The evaluator has an obligation to explain how the impending decision to fire the director could immediately affect the evaluation as well as the community. The Guiding Principles themselves serve as a useful framework for presenting the multilayered consequences of such a decision. They would allow the evaluator to methodically enumerate each impact as it potentially damages the validity of the evaluation process and ultimately its findings.

All of the suggestions discussed in the previous sections can be used here to achieve an evaluation process that deliberately seeks the public welfare. Collectively, these methods support transparency of information, critical multiplism, and a fair hearing of information. Although these approaches can be integrated into an ongoing evaluation, they stand the best chance of successful use if they are introduced at the beginning of the project.

CONCLUSIONS

Conventional wisdom indicates that "the best offense is a good defense." Accordingly, I offer the following suggestions as strategies that might have helped to prevent the sort of problem that occurred in The Folder scenario.

Initially, an evaluator should outline the logic of the evaluation design, the benefits and disadvantages of the approach, the assumptions made, and the consequences that might ensue if assumptions are violated. Such a checklist serves several purposes. First, it can represent a contract, which sets parameters and identifies limitations before the implementation of the evaluation. Second, during the implementation phase, it can serve as a continuous feedback mechanism and filter for guiding evaluation decisions. It allows both the evaluator and client to depersonalize difficult issues and make critical decisions as they relate to standards of Systematic Inquiry. In The Folder scenario, a checklist would have given the client and evaluator a framework for identifying potential ethical issues before the evaluation, and provided a process for addressing emergent issues, such as the difficulties with the director, during the implementation of the project.

Learn the language of stakeholders. This takes time and energy. This learning requires that the participants respect each other's intellectual and social positions and histories. Such an approach could have given The Folder evaluator crucial insights into the community that would inform the evaluation's questions, frame its design and implementation, and alert her to the signs of growing dissatisfaction with the director.

Finally, use your "border space" if you are an evaluator who has knowledge of dominant groups but at the same time lacks the full privileges afforded true insiders. Such individuals have unique advantages when they choose to use their location to investigate power arrangements. Most importantly, they embody a combination of remoteness and concern (Collins, 1986). This dual focus allows the evaluator to ask questions that generate a more informed agenda for social change. This purposeful use of self provides a deeper understanding of how cultural incompetence can occur, is reproduced, and can be challenged.

Centering, driven primarily by a concern for social justice, takes an evaluator to engaged subjectivity and reflexivity, critically reflecting on the impact of the social and historic locations of all stakeholders. Such an orientation helps the evaluator manage the evaluation experience in ways that can lessen the incidence of The Folder-type dilemmas.

REFERENCES

Agar, M. H. (1980). *The professional stranger: An informal introduction to ethnography.* New York: Academic Press.

American Evaluation Association. (2004). *Guiding principles for evaluators* (rev.). Available at *www.eval.org/Publications/GuidingPrinciples.asp.*

Collins, P. H. (1986). Learning from the outsider within: The sociological significance of black feminist thought. *Social Problems, 33,* 14–32.

Cousins, J. B., & Earl, L. M. (1995). (Eds.). *Participatory evaluation in education: Studies in evaluation use and organizational learning.* Bristol, PA: Falmer.

Crenshaw, K. (1989). Forward: Toward a race-conscious pedagogy in legal education. *National Black Law Journal, 11*(1), 1–14.

Datta, L. (1999). The ethics of evaluation neutrality and advocacy. In J. L. Fitzpatrick & M. Morris (Eds.), *Current and emerging ethical challenges in evaluation* (New directions for evaluation, no. 82, pp. 77–88). San Francisco: Jossey-Bass.

Fetterman, D. M. (2000). *Foundations of empowerment evaluation: Step by step.* London: Sage.

Frierson, H. T., Hood, S., & Hughes, G. B. (2002). Strategies that address culturally responsive evaluation. In J. Frechtling (Ed.), *The 2002 user-friendly handbook for project evaluation* (pp. 63–73). Arlington, VA: National Science Foundation.

Greene, J. C. (1988). Communication of results and utilization in participatory program evaluation. *Evaluation and Program Planning, 11,* 341–351.

Guzman, B., & Feria, A. (2002). Community-based organizations and state initiatives: The negotiation process of program evaluation. In R. Mohan, D. Bernstein, & M. Whitsett (Eds.), *Responding to sponsors and stakeholders in complex evaluation environments* (New directions for evaluation, no. 95, pp. 57–72). San Francisco: Jossey-Bass.

House, E. R. (2001). Responsive evaluation (and its influence on deliberative democratic evaluation). In J. C. Greene & T. A. Abma (Eds.), *Responsive evaluation* (New directions for evaluation, no. 92, pp. 23–30). San Francisco: Jossey-Bass.

House, E. R., & Howe, K. R. (1998). The issue of advocacy in evaluations. *American Journal of Evaluation, 19,* 233–236.

Jackson, J. S., Torres, M., Caldwell, C. C., Neighbors, H. W., Nesse, R. M., Taylor, R. J., et al. (2004). The National Survey of American Life: A study of racial, ethnic and cultural influences on mental disorders and mental health. *International Journal of Methods in Psychiatric Research, 13,* 196–207.

Kirkhart, K. E. (1995). Seeking multicultural validity: A postcard from the road. *Evaluation Practice, 16*(1), 1–12.

Mertens, D. M. (1999). Inclusive evaluation: Implications of transformative theory for evaluation. *American Journal of Evaluation, 20,* 1–14.

Patton, M. Q. (1997). *Utilization-focused evaluation: The new century text* (3rd ed.). Thousand Oaks, CA: Sage.

Putnam, H. (1990). *Realism with a human face.* Cambridge, MA: Harvard University Press.

Ryan, K., Greene, J., Lincoln, Y., Mathison, S., & Mertens, D. M. (1998). Advantages and disadvantages of using inclusive evaluation approaches in evaluation practice. *American Journal of Evaluation, 19,* 101–122.

Smith, L. T. (1999). *Decolonizing methodologies: Research and indigenous peoples.* New York: Palgrave.

Stake, R. E. (1975). *Evaluating the arts in education: A responsive approach.* Columbus, OH: Merrill.

Stanley, L., & Wise, S. (1983). *Breaking out: Feminist consciousness and feminist research.* London: Routledge & Kegan Paul.

Thomas, V. G. (2004). Building a contextually responsive evaluation framework: Lessons from working with urban school interventions. In V. G. Thomas & F. I. Stevens (Eds.), *Co-constructing a contextually responsive evaluation framework: The talent development model of school reform* (New directions for evaluation, no. 101, pp. 3–23). San Francisco: Jossey-Bass.

Trochim, W. (1989). An introduction to concept mapping for planning and evaluation. *Evaluation and Program Planning, 12,* 1–16.

■   ■   ■   ■

WHAT IF . . . ?

. . . *in the middle of your meeting with the SNA chairperson, he says, "The board is thinking about firing the director. I know that evaluating his job performance is not one of your responsibilities, but what do you think we should do?"?*

. . . *the SNA has indeed provided the Director with constructive, performance-enhancing feedback, and in your opinion his performance has improved modestly?*

. . . *in your opinion, the director has been doing an excellent job, and you believe that certain influential SNA constituencies are "out to get him"?*

The Folder

Hendricks and davis bring very different perspectives to The Folder case. For davis, the ethical course of action for the evaluator is clear: "The Guiding Principles clearly compel the evaluator to disclose knowledge of her discovery to *all* stakeholders." In sharp contrast, Hendricks believes that the Guiding Principles might not even be relevant to the situation facing the evaluator (cf. Pipes, Holstein, & Aguirre, 2005). Moreover, if they are relevant, he maintains that they could be legitimately viewed as *prohibiting* the evaluator from sharing her discovery with anyone other than the SNA chairperson. Hendricks does allow that the professional experience of the evaluator might intersect with the circumstances of the scenario in a manner whereby the Guiding Principles would permit, and perhaps even encourage (but *not* require), the evaluator to lobby both the SNA chairperson and the foundation for a reconsideration of the apparent plan to terminate the director. Of course, this response falls far short of approaching "all stakeholders" with the information, as davis recommends.

What are we to make of these differences? Well, davis has applied what Hendricks would call a "liberal" perspective to the scenario. That is, she emphasizes the implications for the evaluation and its stakeholders of how the Governing Board deals with the director's performance. This sets the stage for the evaluator adopting a more proactive strategy for handling her discovery than would otherwise be appropriate. That being said, there is still no escaping the fact that davis sees the evaluator as having an ethical mandate in The Folder case that is much stronger, and more expansive, than Hendricks seems to think is warranted, even under liberal assumptions.

Hendricks's and davis's analyses differ in at least one other important way. For davis, an in-depth understanding of the community context within which the evaluation is taking place (centering) is critical to developing an ethical, effective response to the scenario. These sorts of contextual details (community demographics, history, culture) play no direct role in Hendricks's discussion of how the evaluator should act. Rather, the key factors he considers are the nature of the evaluation (Is performance appraisal involved?) and the evaluator's work experience (How relevant is this experience to the current dilemma?).

One might argue that, in The Folder scenario, the primary influence of the contextual dimensions stressed by davis is on the *form* or *style* of the evaluator's reaction to the ethical problem rather than on the fundamental *substance* of that reaction. Asserting that the "Guiding Principles clearly compel the evaluator to disclose knowledge of her discovery to *all* stakeholders" does not leave much "wiggle room" for variations in community culture and demographics to alter one's basic ethical responsibility.

Against this background, the contrasting analyses of our two commentators remind us of at least two crucial tasks that all evaluators face: (1) determining the relevance of multiple contextual factors when encountering an ethical challenge in a particular evaluation project, and (2) judging the substantive and stylistic implications of that relevance for upholding the Guiding Principles. As The Folder case vividly demonstrates, when different evaluators engage in these tasks, the possibility exists that different conclusions will be reached. To what extent do you think Hendricks and davis have adequately justified their analyses? How would you justify yours?

REFERENCE

Pipes, R. B., Holstein, J. E., & Aguirre, M. G. (2005). Examining the personal-professional distinction: Ethics codes and the difficulty of drawing a boundary. *American Psychologist, 60,* 325–334.

Hideout

For the past month you have been conducting confidential interviews at several halfway houses where selected male offenders serve the last 6 months of their prison sentences. Operated by a private, not-for-profit agency largely funded by the state's Department of Corrections, the halfway houses' purpose is to facilitate offenders' reintegration into the community. The department has hired you, an external evaluator, to carry out a process evaluation focusing on participants' experiences in the program.

This afternoon you interviewed a 22-year-old former gang member, who, in the course of reflecting on his gang-related activities, mentioned a specific location in the community where, according to him, the gang stores weapons and illegal drugs. Some of the weapons are sold, and others are used by the gang members themselves in the commission of crimes. Most of the drugs are sold on the street.

After the interview you wonder if you should do anything with this information. There is no doubt that law enforcement officials would enthusiastically welcome news about the whereabouts of this contraband, especially in view of the media attention that a recent crime wave, attributed to the gang, has received. And it is certainly true that one less illegal gun on the street is one less gun that can be used to wound or kill someone. That's clearly relevant to the public good.

On the other hand, you are under no legal obligation to reveal what you have been told. And sharing what you know with the police would certainly violate the confidentiality agreement you have with your interviewees in this study. Indeed, there is a chance, although not necessarily a high-probability one, that the young man in question would be put in harm's way if you go to the authorities, despite your best efforts to protect his identity. Do the benefits of seizing the weapons and drugs outweigh the risks to which your "informant" is exposed? And what about your credibility as a researcher if word gets out that you breached confidentiality? To put it mildly, interviewees are likely to be very wary of you, and perhaps other evaluators, in the future ("Don't believe evaluators' promises!"). Do you have the right to take an action that might taint not only your reputation but theirs as well?

You're mulling over all of this as you purchase a copy of the local paper on the way home. The lead story reports the fatal shooting of an innocent bystander in a gang-related incident.

QUESTIONS TO CONSIDER

1. Can Hendricks's life-experience/evaluation-experience analysis be applied to this case in the same way that it was to The Folder case?

2. If you were 100% confident that the interviewee was providing you with accurate information about the location of the contraband, would it make a difference in how you respond in this situation? Why or why not?

3. What if you were absolutely sure that the interviewee's identity could be protected? Would that belief affect your decision?

4. Should the impact of your action on the overall reputation of evaluators play a role in your response to this case?

5. In the event that you chose *not* to go to law enforcement officials with what you've been told, is there *anyone* you would share the information with?

CHAPTER FIVE

Data Analysis and Interpretation

Knock, Knock, What's There?

Well, the data are in, and now a contentious discussion is taking place among the members of the evaluation team you lead. The team had employed a strong randomized design to assess the impact of a complex, comprehensive program to increase conservation practices among homeowners in a large northeastern city, as measured by consumption indicators on electric, gas, and water bills. Viewed through the lens of traditional levels of statistical significance, the program does not appear to have made a difference. Although there are some trends in the data suggesting the efficacy of the intervention, in no instance is a difference between the experimental and control groups significant at the .05 level. The differences that do exist occasionally reach a significance level of .10. These overall findings are robust, withstanding a variety of subgroup analyses. Given the large number of households participating in the study, this doesn't seem to be a case in which weak results can be attributed to small sample size.

As far as two members of your team are concerned, this is a "cut-and-dry case of *no effect*." "Let's face facts," Jake asserts, "the program doesn't work. We've conducted a well-designed study and are on solid methodological ground. We shouldn't let ourselves be seduced by a few *p* < .10s scattered here and there throughout the results. It's not often that we're in a position to offer a definitive interpretation of a program's effectiveness, given the compromised designs we so often have to work with. This is no time to get cold feet. This is an expensive intervention that consumes resources that could be put to better use."

Marjorie and Tim do not find Jake's argument convincing. "I disagree that this is a cut-and-dry case," Marjorie responds. "Virtually every observed difference between the experimental and control groups, and there are a fair number, favors the experimental group. Don't you think that means something? You don't want us to be seduced by $p < .10$, but should we be held hostage by blind allegiance to a $p < .05$ significance level? A blanket interpretation of *no effect* just doesn't seem to be warranted in this situation. A strong design gives one the *opportunity* to come to a definitive conclusion, but only if the data justify it. If we were studying a drug used to treat a deadly disease, would you be so quick to dismiss these results as definitive evidence of *no effect*? We have an ethical responsibility here to be sensitive to the patterns we see in the data. You're oversimplifying our choice of interpretation, reducing it to a dichotomous decision. It doesn't need to be that, and it shouldn't be that."

Jake exclaims, "Have you lost your mind? The only pattern I see in these results tells me that the intervention lacks the potency to generate a substantive change in the behavior of program participants. What's unethical is offering false hope to program developers, funders, and—in the medical example you give—patients, when the data provide you with so little support, as they do in this case. There isn't one difference at the $p < .05$ level, Marjorie, *not one*. And not enough differences at the $p < .10$ level to make me comfortable that we're not just capitalizing on chance. Do you really want to give everybody a set of rose-colored glasses to look at these findings with? Would that represent doing the right thing as a professional evaluator? I don't think so."

Jake turns to you. "You're the Principal Investigator on this project. It's your interpretation that will end up being shared with our stakeholders. What are you going to do?"

C O M M E N T A R Y

What's There: Confidence or Competence?

Leslie J. Cooksy

As the leader of the team that evaluated a resource conservation program in a large city in the northeastern United States, I am faced with a conflict among my colleagues about how to interpret the results of our analyses. With a randomized design, we had hoped to provide a strong test of the presence, direction, and size of an effect. The conflict centers on the reporting of results that are not statistically significant at a .05 level. Jake argues that we should not report results that do not meet a standard of $p \leq .05$. Marjorie disagrees; she suggests that the overall pattern of results is positive and worth reporting.

The difference of opinion in how to proceed reflects differences in how the two evaluators were trained. Whereas Jake comes from a traditional social science research program that emphasizes quantitative methods, Marjorie is a generalist evaluator, with a strong academic background in evaluation theory and design. Their different skills and perspectives reflect the diversity of the evaluation community, a diversity that is recognized in many statements of the primary professional organization of evaluators in the United States, the American Evaluation Association (AEA). One place where the diversity of evaluation is explicitly addressed is in the preface to AEA's Guiding Principles for Evaluators, which refers to "differences in training, experience, and work settings" and in "perceptions about the primary purpose of evaluation" (American Evaluation Association, 2004, Preface-B). While accepting diversity in these dimensions of the profession, the Guiding Principles state that evaluators are united by a common aspiration "to construct and provide the best possible information that might bear on the value of whatever is being evaluated" (Preface-B). Unfortunately, as Marjorie's and Jake's disagreement indicates, different evaluators may have conflicting opinions about what constitutes the "best possible information." As the leader of the evaluation of the conservation program, it is up to me to decide what information is appropriate to report in this situation. I agree with Marjorie that the data can be interpreted and reported in a way that is useful and informative beyond a simple conclusion of "not effective" based on p values of greater than .05.

My decision is based on my own training and experience as an evaluator, which has been guided by the logic of pattern matching: the comparison of observed patterns in the data with anticipated theoretical patterns (Shadish, Cook, & Campbell, 2002; Trochim, 1985). The way that Jake was using statistical significance testing is not compatible with a pattern-matching approach. Before announcing my decision to the team, however, I first use the Guiding Principles to review the implications of our data analysis and interpretation. The results of this review are presented in the next section. Then, my prescription for analyzing, interpreting, and reporting the evaluation results will be described. The commentary concludes with the doubts that linger in my mind after I have made my decision.

ETHICAL ISSUES IN THE CASE
OF THE CONSERVATION PROGRAM EVALUATION

At first glance, statistical significance testing may seem to be an issue primarily related to the Guiding Principles of Systematic Inquiry and Competence. Reviewing the evaluation for consistency with the Systematic Inquiry principle, one wants to know the strength of the design, the size and representativeness of the sample, the reliability and validity of the measurement tools, and the appropriateness of the statistical tests given the evaluation design, sample, and type and quality of the data. The ability to get these elements right is based on the competence of the evaluation team: Does it have the skills needed to design and conduct the evaluation and, in this case, specifically to choose the right significance tests and interpret them correctly? The link between Systematic Inquiry and Competence and the other Guiding Principles relates to what Fish (1993), in describing the pitfalls of significance testing in evaluation, called the "special moral as well as scientific obligations" of the evaluator (p. 2). The moral obligations are created by the fact that inappropriate methods "may result in an unwarranted termination of program funds, staff dismissals, or a general climate of hostility to a deserving program" (Fish, 1993, p. 2). Thus, analysis decisions also relate to the principles of Honesty/Integrity, Respect for People, and Responsibilities for General and Public Welfare.

Systematic Inquiry

In general, the evaluation has been consistent with the principle of Systematic Inquiry. The randomized design, although not universally endorsed (e.g., Guba & Lincoln, 1989; Pawson & Tilley, 1997), is upheld by many as the best means of discovering whether an intervention has caused an observed effect (e.g., Boruch, 1997; Shadish et al., 2002). Note, however, that the proponents of randomized design recognize that it is not appropriate in all circumstances (Boruch, 2005; Mark, Henry, & Julnes, 2000; Shadish, Cook, & Campbell, 2002). The conservation program evaluation met the five criteria articulated by Boruch (2005) defining when a randomized design is appropriate. First, it addresses a serious problem: the need for energy conservation; resource use in the United States continues to increase; natural resources, especially energy resources, continue to decrease; and political decisions based on the country's energy needs have long-range implications for our relationships with other nations around the globe. Second, there is genuine uncertainty about how to deal with the problem: Although many localities offer energy and water conservation incentives and benefits, these interventions have not been systematically evaluated. So, for example, it is unknown whether the households that take a tax break for adding insulation to their attics would have added the insulation without the tax breaks because of a preexisting interest in energy conservation. Thus, there is a real opportunity for a randomized trial to inform future policy on effective ways of encouraging resource conservation. Third, alternative evaluation designs are unlikely to be as defensible in the policy arena as the randomized design. Fourth, there is reason to believe that the results will be used: Politicians from the mayor of the city participating in the study to the president of the United States are seeking ways to diminish the public's use of finite energy resources. Credible information on a serious problem that has high visibility in national debates is likely to be used to contribute to the debate (Weiss & Bucuvalas, 1981). Finally, random assignment is ethically appropriate in this case: No participant in the study was denied gas, electricity, or water resources; members of both experimental and control groups received information on conservation practices; and there were not enough resources to provide the intervention to everyone who was interested. In addition, an advisory group convened by the program designers and including community members, experts, and others could not identify any likely risks to participating in the study for either the treatment or control groups.

The design was not only well chosen, it was also well implemented. The team diligently documented any changes in the experimental and control groups so that issues such as treatment diffusion or differential attrition could be controlled in the analysis (Shadish et al.,

2002). The dependent variables of electric, gas, and water consumption were measured directly and with a high degree of reliability by the meter readings reported on the utility bills of the households participating in the study. With household bills as the source of data, we were able to collect multiple pretests and posttests so that seasonal cycles could be controlled for.

Although the evaluation design and implementation were generally quite strong, the sample was a weakness. Like many true experiments, the participants are not a random sample of the population of interest (households in the Northeast United States). Instead, they are the households that responded to a request for volunteers to participate in the evaluation. In other words, simply by agreeing to participate in the study, these households are expressing some interest in the idea of conservation. If the sample consists of people already motivated to conserve resources, the effects of the program may be more difficult to detect because both treatment and control groups may already be seeking ways to limit their use of electricity, gas, and water. In addition, despite the large sample size mentioned in the case description, the sample is not as large as needed to detect relatively small treatment effects. When negotiating with our clients about the methodology and costs of the study, we showed them the sample size required to detect small treatment effects that had been estimated by our power analysis. The clients said that, given the cost of obtaining such a large sample, we would have to have fewer participants. With the strengths of the other elements of the design and the size of the effect anticipated by the program designers, we thought that our design was likely to be sufficiently sensitive, even with a smaller sample, to keep us from committing a Type II error (i.e., claiming no effect when, in fact, there is one).

So, with a strong design, low measurement error, and a sample that is large enough to detect at least moderate effects, the remaining element of inquiry that needs to be systematic is the data analysis. As the scenario describes, Jake's approach is to compare the means of the treatment and control groups, calculate the p value, and decide whether or not there is a treatment effect based on whether the p value is less than or greater than .05. Although typical, this strategy is not appropriate. From at least as early as 1960, researchers in the social sciences have questioned the value of tests of statistical significance for both technical and philosophical reasons (e.g., Carver, 1978; Fish, 1993; Meehl, 1991; Rozeboom, 1960). The conservation program evaluation suffered from one of the technical problems raised by critics of the use of statistical significance testing: The households participating in the study were not randomly selected from the population, which is a violation of the assumptions for the tests being used. When Marjorie raised this issue with Jake, he gave the answer he had learned from his professor: "Oh, forget about that, most significance tests are robust against violations of the assumptions." Marjorie, a purist, simply pursed her lips and reminded herself that Jake was supposed to be the expert.

Although concerned with technical problems, opponents of statistical significance testing are often more disturbed by the *theoretical* problems posed by the use of statistical significance tests to accept or reject hypotheses (Carver, 1978; Fish, 1993; Meehl, 1991; Rozeboom, 1960; Shadish et al., 2002). Hubbard and Armstrong (2005) identified some of the most common misinterpretations of the outcomes of significance tests: "Such tests are erroneously believed to indicate the probability that (1) the results occurred because of chance, (2) the results will replicate, (3) the alternative hypothesis is true, (4) the results will generalize, and (5) the results are substantively significant" (Hubbard & Armstrong, 2005, pp. 1–2). Given the opportunities for misinterpretation, the choice and interpretation of statistical tests are two of the keys to ensuring that this evaluation was conducted in a manner consistent with the principle of Systematic Inquiry. I am convinced that we can learn more from the results of the evaluation than whether or not the null hypothesis of no effect should be rejected, as Jake is recommending.

Competence

The evaluation team had been somewhat hastily put together once the contract for the evaluation was finally signed. Marjorie and Jake are junior staff, with doctoral degrees in relevant fields and good recommendations from their professors but lacking much experience in evaluation practice. Tim has more experience with evaluation and was our "people person," in charge of randomly assigning participants, coordinating the interviewer training, and interacting with the client. Although I felt that I had a capable team, there were potential gaps in competence. The one that became an issue was a lack of sophistication about statistical tests.

Although Jake was our designated analyst, his eagerness to use the p value as a decision tool indicates a superficial knowledge of the application of statistical significance testing in evaluation. As the team leader, I was concerned that I had failed to follow the Competence principle of ensuring that the evaluation team had all the skills needed to undertake the evaluation. Although not a statistician myself, I knew that the debate about the value of statistical significance testing had mostly resolved itself against using a preestablished level for Type I error (α) to decide whether to accept or reject a hypothesis of no effect. Instead, effect size estimates, with 95% confidence intervals, and exact p values, the measure of "the proportion of the time that we can expect to find mean differences as large as or larger than the particular sized difference we get when we are sampling from the same population assumed under the null hypothesis" (Carver, 1978, p. 382), should be reported (Shadish et al., 2002).[1] After a review of my design and statistics texts and discussion with some colleagues, I decide that we should use the pretest data in analyses of covariance (ANCOVAs), after checking for violations of the assumptions particular to ANCOVA, to control for any preintervention differences between the experimental and control groups and, in turn, increase the sensitivity of the analysis (Lipsey, 1990).

Although I am confident about not employing the .05 probability of a Type I error as the sole indicator of the meaningfulness of the data, I know that deciding against using the .05 standard to determine what results to report in the conservation evaluation will open up the study to criticisms in some circles. The vast number of evaluators and other social scientists who have been trained like Jake to worship the .05 standard are likely to question whether we have truly adhered to the highest technical standards if we use other criteria for determining the value of the information. As I describe later, I hope to forestall that criticism when the results are reported.

Integrity/Honesty

The main way that the scenario engages the Integrity/Honesty principle is in relation to the guidance that "if evaluators determine that certain procedures or activities are likely to produce misleading evaluative information or conclusions, they have the responsibility to communicate their concerns and the reasons for them" (American Evaluation Association, 2004, Principle C-6). Other advice provided by the principle, such as avoiding conflict of interest and communicating clearly about the scope, costs and limitations of the evaluation, or changes in the evaluation plan, have been followed. However, if questions are raised about the competence of the team's analysis of results, and the results themselves are considered by some to be misleading, then questions may be raised about our integrity. Will presenting results that are informative but not decisive be dishonest? As with the question about competence, I feel that potential attacks on our integrity can be warded off with clear and informative reporting.

Respect for People

The principle of Respect for People is invoked by the ethical issues associated with randomized designs in which resources or services may be denied to participants. In this case, as discussed in the rationale for using an experimental design, there is genuine uncertainty about whether the intervention is beneficial and general agreement that the risks of assignment to either the intervention or control group are minimal. However, the question of the choice of statistical test and interpretation of results raises another Respect for People concern. When we ask individuals to participate in a study, obtain personal information about their habits (use of electricity, gas, and water in this case), and monitor the extent to which they received the intervention, we have an obligation to use that information to the fullest so that their time and goodwill are not wasted. One of the ways we compensate those who provide data is by analyzing the data appropriately and reporting it clearly so that it can have the widest possible use.

Sometimes our reporting of results is a cautionary tale; in other words, our report is less informative about a program's results than about difficulties in evaluating such a program. But even if the evaluation cannot provide findings that can be used to understand, manage, or make policy about a program, it should provide information about the practice of evaluation. One of the ways that we respect evaluation participants is by discovering what lessons can be appropriately and usefully gleaned from the evaluation and communicating them to the individuals who can use them.

Responsibilities for General and Public Welfare

One reason to care so much about whether and how to use statistical significance testing is that our conclusions about the conservation program are likely to be influential. The effects of the intervention really are unknown and, because of the political implications of our reliance on foreign energy sources, the debate about the results is likely to be contentious. A strong design in a politically contentious debate can be influential (Boruch, 1997; Weiss & Bucuvalas, 1981). As a result, analyzing and interpreting the data correctly are not just relevant to the principle of Competence but also to Responsibilities for General and Public Welfare.

Is Jake right? Is the conservation program "an expensive intervention that consumes resources that could be put to better use"? Will our evaluation, if it suggests otherwise, be promoting the inefficient and ineffective use of public money? On the other hand, if this program does have some redeeming features that are not revealed by the statistical tests, a rush to judge it as unsalvageable could result not only in wasted time and money but in the wasting of the resources that need to be conserved. On the basis of our responsibility to the public and to our clients, I know that the question we have to answer is not "Was the program effective?" but rather "What did we learn about the program from this evaluation?"

GUIDED BY PRINCIPLES

To answer the question about what we learned concerning the conservation program, we have to review what previous evaluations of similar conservation programs have shown and what pattern of effects the program designers anticipated based on their knowledge of resource consumption patterns and approaches to changing them. This information had been gathered at the beginning of the evaluation but had not yet been used to inform the analysis. Using it to inform the analysis is expected to increase the sensitivity of the design to possible treatment effects and to test the congruence of the observed pattern with the theoretical pattern, a better strategy than using simpler tests of difference between the treatment and control groups' mean consumption of electricity, gas, and water. In addition, the previous subgroup comparisons will be reconsidered to see how the results compare with those found in evaluations of similar programs. Finally, to meet our responsibility to the public welfare, we have to go beyond just doing a better job of analyzing the data and placing it in the context of prior research. We have to report the findings in ways that are credible, accessible, and, ideally, educational about the use of statistical tests. This section outlines both the analysis and reporting plans that my team and I develop, following the decision that Jake's statistical tests are not an appropriate approach to interpreting the results.

Design Sensitivity and Pattern Matching

As reported earlier, we were already planning to increase our confidence in any treatment effects observed by using ANCOVA to account for between-group differences in the pretest data. Increasing design sensitivity is also the purpose behind reviewing previous evaluations of similar conservation programs and mapping the anticipated pattern of effects. A narrative review of relevant evaluations can help identify likely relationships among variables (Shadish et al., 2002). Similarly, a structured conceptualization method can help the program developers articulate their local program theory, especially the pattern of relationships among outcome variables that they would expect to see based on their experience and knowledge (Mark, 1990; Trochim, 1985, 1989b). Divergent results for different sectors of the population are another kind of pattern that can be identified (Mark, 1990). Although the simplicity of the true experiment as a means of ruling out plausible alternative hypotheses is one of its great virtues, analyzing the data for congruence with a theoretical pattern of results increases the practical value of the evaluation for its potential audiences. For example, if the analyses show that the treatment effect is larger for water conservation than for electricity, the program may be considered more applicable to a drought-stricken part of the country than for the cold and rainy Northeast. Similarly, larger treatment effects for people in the Southeast part of the city than for those in the Northwest could generate ideas for how to target the intervention more effectively in the future.

Although this approach could greatly strengthen the sensitivity of the design to any effects and increase its practical utility, it has problems. As Shadish et al. (2002) note, statistical tests of the overall fit of the data to the hypothesized pattern are required, and these are not as well developed or understood as are comparisons of the means of treatment and control groups. Because we are running multiple statistical tests (especially since Jake has already compared group means), we also need to address the criticism that we have been fishing for more interesting results. I prefer the Bonferroni correction for multiple tests (Snedecor & Cochran, 1980; Shadish et al., 2002). It is conservative, so the resulting p values are less likely to instill confidence in the findings, but it also demonstrates our concern for not overstating a case that the program is effective. Because we will report effect size, confidence intervals, and p values instead of whether comparisons of group means were statistically significant based on a predetermined alpha, the audience will be able to make their own judgment of whether we have been too conservative.

Reporting Results

Reporting is key to completing this evaluation in a way that is consistent with the Guiding Principles. Four of the five Guiding Principles place great emphasis on evaluation reporting. For Systematic Inquiry, evaluators should "make clear the limitations of an evaluation and its results" (American Evaluation Association, 2004, Principle A-3). For Integrity/Honesty, "evaluators should not misrepresent their procedures, data or findings" (Principle C-5). The principle of Respect for People instructs that "evaluators should conduct the evaluation and communicate its results in a way that clearly respects the stakeholders' dignity and self-worth" (Principle D-4). For Responsibilities for General and Public Welfare, "evaluators should strive to present results clearly and simply so that clients and other stakeholders can easily understand the evaluation process and results" (Principle E-3).

With a large study, somewhat complex analyses, and ambiguous results, reporting appropriately and clearly is quite a chore. We have the additional burden of communicating our rationale for not using $p \leq .05$ as a standard for determining whether a treatment effect has been observed, so that readers understand that we have used appropriate technical standards. At the same time that we need to be explicit about our technical choices, we also have to present our results in a way that is clear about their limitations without undercutting any lessons that can be learned.

Our plan is to first show treatment effect sizes for the different kinds of resources (gas, electricity, and water) and confidence intervals using error bars, so that the audience has a picture of how uncertain the results are. Once the reader understands the potential error of the estimated treatment effects, the pattern of effect sizes will be visually presented next to a matching visual display of the hypothesized patterns of conservation. A similar approach would be used to show differences between subgroups. For each display of data, a clear explanation of the likely practical significance of the results will be provided in layperson's terms. Those with more technical interest and sophistication will be directed to detailed appendices. In both places, the limitations of the data and the ambiguity of some of the results will be highlighted. By the same token, results that seem promising will also be identified. To acknowledge the contributions of the households that participated in the study, each will be sent a thank you letter providing a brief summary of the results and describing how to get the more detailed report.

Through the combination of thoughtful analyses and audience-friendly presentation, I expect that the evaluation will yield more than Jake's conclusion of "no effect" could. If nothing else, I'll know that we will have provided valuable information for other evaluators to use in planning future studies or including our evaluation in a meta-analysis.

CONFUSION ABOUT COMPETENCE

The case of the conservation program evaluation is based on the question, How should the data be analyzed and interpreted? Although the principles of Honesty/Integrity, Respect for People, and Responsibilities for General and Public Welfare are certainly involved, this question is fundamentally an issue of evaluator (or evaluation team) competence. The Systematic Inquiry principle implies some understanding of what the "highest technical standards" are for a given method. If we know what these standards are, it is then possible to assess how close we have come to meeting them. However, the conservation program case illustrates that even in what seems at first to be a narrow and clear-cut subject—statistical significance testing—there can be disagreement about what appropriate practices are. If, as evaluators, we are indeed united in our goal of constructing and providing "the best possible information that might bear on the value of whatever is being evaluated" (American Evaluation Association, 2004, Preface-B), should we not have some common understanding of what "best possible" looks like for a given approach to evaluation? Specifically, in this instance, shouldn't Jake, Marjorie, and I share an understanding concerning the appropriate analysis?

The answer, of course, is yes, and the good news is that the experts know what the analysis options are and which should be chosen given specific conditions. So then the question becomes, Why was there disagreement? Here is Jake, PhD in hand, recommended by his professors, member of an evaluation team with a big contract, confident in his knowledge of quantitative analysis. Here am I, with almost two decades of experience as a professional evaluator, much of it spent learning how much there will always be that I do not know, trying to do an honest and competent job. Jake is more confident than competent. My competence is manifest in a combination of lack of confidence about the particulars of certain tasks in evaluation built on a foundation of confidence that *I know the areas in which I need to seek outside help.* It is counterintuitive, but I attribute my relative lack of confidence to the quality of my training and the diversity of my experience. My training taught me to ask the question, How can I be wrong in making a claim of knowledge about a program? My experience has shown me the many ways it is possible to be wrong. Jake was never taught to ask how he could be wrong. He was only taught what was "right." From my perspective, this gave Jake an inappropriate confidence in his own competence.

The Competence principle says that "evaluators should practice within the limits of their professional training and competence" (American Evaluation Association, 2004, Principle B-3) and that "evaluators should continually seek to maintain and improve their competencies, in order to provide the highest level of performance in their evaluations" (Principle B-4). These both imply that evaluators know what the limits of their competence are. Perhaps an additional clause should be added: "Evaluators should rarely assume that they know the limits of their competence." Even as I judge Jake to be overconfident, I have to question my own confidence that I, in fact, know when I need to seek the advice of experts. As evaluators, we should be asking of ourselves, not just of the claims that we make for programs; How might we be wrong?

NOTE

1. Hubbard and Armstrong (2005) describe the distinction between Fisher's p value and the Neyman–Pearson (N-P) α in hypothesis testing, stating that, for N-P, "the specific value of p itself is irrelevant and should not be reported. In the N-P decision model the researcher can only say whether or not a result fell in the rejection region, but not where it fell" (p. 6).

REFERENCES

American Evaluation Association. (2004). *Guiding principles for evaluators* (rev.). Available at *www.eval.org/Publications/GuidingPrinciples.asp.*

Bickman, L. (Ed.). (1990). *Advances in program theory* (New directions for program evaluation, no. 47). San Francisco: Jossey-Bass.

Boruch, R. F. (1997). *Randomized field experiments for planning and evaluation: A practical guide.* Thousand Oaks, CA: Sage.

Boruch, R. F. (2005). Comments on "Use of randomization in the evaluation of development effectiveness." In G. K. Pitman, O. N. Feinstein, & G. K. Ingram (Eds.), *World Bank series on evaluation and development: Vol. 7. Evaluating development effectiveness* (pp. 232–239). New Brunswick, NJ: Transaction.

Carver, R. P. (1978). The case against statistical significance testing. *Harvard Educational Review, 48,* 378–399.

Fish, L. (1993, November). *A critique of parametric hypothesis testing in educational research and evaluation.* Paper presented at the annual meeting of the American Evaluation Association, Dallas, TX.

Guba, E. G., & Lincoln, Y. S. (1989). *Fourth generation evaluation.* Newbury Park, CA: Sage.

Hubbard, R., & Armstrong, J. S. (2005). *Why we don't really know what "statistical significance" means: A major educational failure.* Retrieved March 6, 2006, from *marketing.wharton.upenn.edu/ideas/pdf/armstrong/StatisticalSignificance.pdf.*

Lipsey, M. W. (1990). *Design sensitivity: Statistical power for experimental research.* Newbury Park, CA: Sage.

Mark, M. M. (1990). From program theory to tests of program theory. In L. Bickman (Ed.), *Advances in program theory* (New directions for program evaluation, no. 47, pp. 37–51). San Francisco: Jossey-Bass.

Mark, M. M., Henry, G. T., & Julnes, G. (2000). *Evaluation: An integrated framework for understanding, guiding, and improving policies and programs.* San Francisco: Jossey-Bass.

Meehl, P. E. (1991). Theoretical risks and tabular asterisks: Sir Karl, Sir Ronald and the slow progress of soft psychology. In C. A. Anderson & K. Gunderson (Eds.), *Paul E. Meehl: Selected philosophical and methodological papers* (pp. 1–43). Minneapolis: University of Minnesota Press.

Pawson, R., & Tilley, N. (1997). *Realistic evaluation.* London: Sage.

Rozeboom, W. W. (1960). The fallacy of the null-hypothesis significance test. *Psychological Bulletin, 57,* 416–428.

Shadish, W. R., Cook, T. D., & Campbell, D. T. (2002). *Experimental and quasi-experimental designs for generalized causal inference.* Boston: Houghton Mifflin.

Snedecor, G. W., & Cochran, W. G. (1980). *Statistical methods* (7th ed.). Ames: Iowa State University Press.

Trochim, W. M. K. (1985). Pattern matching, validity, and conceptualization in program evaluation. *Evaluation Review, 9,* 575-604.

Trochim, W. (1989a). Concept mapping: Soft science or hard art? *Evaluation and Program Planning, 12,* 87–110.

Trochim, W. M. K. (1989b). Outcome pattern matching and program theory. *Evaluation and Program Planning, 12,* 355–366.

Weiss, C. H., & Bucuvalas, M. J. (1981). Truth tests and utility tests: Decision-makers' frame of reference for social science research. In H. E. Freeman & M. A. Solomon (Eds.), *Evaluation studies review annual* (Vol. 6, pp. 695–706). Beverly Hills, CA: Sage.

Interpreting Effects

William R. Shadish

Many evaluators have had the experience of devoting large amounts of time and resources to evaluating the effects of an intervention, only to find disappointingly small or nonsignificant effects. Such results often displease nearly everyone. The program funders and implementers are disappointed that all their time, effort, and money may not have had the payoff that they wished. The funders of the evaluation almost never hope for null effects because they are usually committed to finding solutions to problems. Policy stakeholders may find it difficult to accept that yet one more hoped-for solution has failed. The evaluator may fear that none of these constituencies will ever seek him or her out again for a contract. So the pressure to find positive results can be quite intense.

In the present case, the investigators are facing this dilemma. By the conventional significance level of $p < .05$, their study yielded no effect. All but the most detached observers would probably admit to at least a tinge of disappointment and would likely be having exactly the same discussion as the investigators. After all, $p < .05$ is just a human creation: Sir Ronald Fisher (1926, p. 504) suggested that number in a somewhat offhand fashion when speculating about how many times we would be willing to say an agricultural intervention works when it really doesn't. But why be rigid about it? As Rosnow and Rosenthal (1989) assert, "Surely God loves the .06 nearly as much as the .05" (p. 1277).

ETHICAL ISSUES

The Guiding Principle of Systematic Inquiry states that "evaluators should adhere to the highest technical standards appropriate to the methods they use" (American Evaluation Association, 2004, Principle A-1). Let us assume that this evaluation had a trivial amount of attrition, that randomization was well implemented, and that the data met all the relevant assumptions (e.g., normality, independence) required by the appropriate statistical tests. If so, then the most salient technical feature of this study that remains unclear is whether the researchers made any correction at all for the multiple outcomes they tested. If not—and it does not seem likely given the description of the case— their dilemma may be greatly reduced. If the investigators did, say, 10 significance tests on outcome variables, then a Bonferroni correction would require significance at $p < .005$ if the outcomes were un- correlated and $p < .01$ if the outcomes were correlated $r = .40$. In either case, the reported results do not come close to that more rigorous stan- dard. This makes the intervention look even less effective.

Good technical work in field experimentation increasingly relies on effect sizes as much as it does on significance levels. This does not just mean effect sizes as expressed in statistics like the standardized mean difference or the correlation coefficient. It can also mean effect sizes expressed in the number of dollars saved, a metric that policy- makers intuitively understand. A competent power analysis done dur- ing the design of the study would presumably have considered that economic metric in establishing the minimum statistical effect size of policy interest, but competent power analyses are few and far between in most evaluations. Too often investigators rely on facile rules of thumb like Cohen's standard that $d = .20$ is a small effect and power their studies accordingly, without ever connecting $d = .20$ to other meaningful metrics like dollars. If an effect of $d = .05$ could result in savings of billions of dollars in energy costs, however, that is certainly policy relevant.

What about the alpha level of .05? After all, the Systematic Inquiry principle says that "evaluators should discuss in a contextually appro- priate way those values, assumptions, theories, methods, results, and analyses significantly affecting the interpretation of the evaluative findings" (American Evaluation Association, 2004, Principle A-3). One of those assumptions is the alpha level we choose, because it expresses an underlying value about the risks we are willing to take in being right or wrong in claiming that a program works. That risk level may vary by context, a point also addressed by the principle of Respect for People, which states that "evaluators should seek a comprehensive understanding of the important contextual elements of the evaluation. Contextual factors that may influence the results of a study include geographic location, timing, political and social climate, economic con- ditions, and other relevant activities in progress at the same time" (Principle D-1).

To illustrate, one can imagine two quite different contexts in which this study might have occurred. In the first, the nation is in an energy crisis that looks to be prolonged, there are no good alternative programs on the drawing board that could affect energy consumption, and even the tiniest of energy savings could result in billions of dollars of savings. In this context, policymakers might be willing to consider further the intervention that was studied, arguing that they would be amenable to taking a somewhat increased risk of being wrong about this intervention given that it has some promise. In the alternative context, this evaluation was just part of a routine program of work investigating potential solutions, many more solutions are on the drawing board or perhaps even available already, and the savings from this program are widely understood to be minimal. This scenario provides little reason for increasing our risk level by going with an alpha level such as .10. Notice that this analysis is also relevant to the Guiding Principle of Responsibilities for General and Public Welfare, which speaks to the evaluator's responsibility to consider the public good.

Finally, these investigators fall into the trap of taking one study too seriously. Policy decisions are rarely made on the basis of one study. Indeed, those decisions are rarely made on the basis of even a review of many studies on the topic, although such reviews are (and should be) more influential than single studies in shaping policy. So, when Jake turns to the principal investigator (PI) and asks what the PI is going to do, the PI might well respond, "Relax!"

Are the Guiding Principles adequate to analyze this case? Probably, given the proviso that they are intentionally couched in very general terms. Clearly, the details I have discussed here about what constitutes "the highest technical standards" could not possibly be detailed in the Guiding Principles for this study or for studies using other methodologies. Hence, this case illustrates the need for more technically oriented guidelines that are exemplified in, say, the Program Evaluation Standards (Joint Committee on Standards for Educational Evaluation, 1994) as well as the ultimate need to appeal to methodological experts whose knowledge and experience best equip them to identify potential failures to meet high technical standards.

WHAT WOULD I DO NOW?

First, I would report the results using both raw and Bonferroni-adjusted probability levels and describe the appropriateness of the latter in most cases. Second, I would report effect size data with particular attention to the number of dollars that might be saved given the statistical effect size observed in the study. Third, my discussion of the results would highlight their place in the overall context of previous research. This study is not likely to be the only one ever to have been done on the topic. My interpretation will be affected by how the results of the present study fit into that past literature in terms of whether these results are (1) consistent with past findings or (2) an anomaly in a literature that usually reports either stronger or weaker effects. In the former case, with a literature full of borderline $p < .10$ effects that are all in the direction of the intended effect, I would strongly suspect that the entire literature suffers from statistical power problems. My solution might well be to conduct a meta-analysis of the literature because this would increase the likelihood that I would find a significant effect if it is there. In the latter case, in which the present result is an anomaly, much depends on the direction of the anomaly. If my evaluation shows the strongest findings in a sea of otherwise null effects, I would quite likely draw discouraging conclusions about the kinds of interventions this study represents. If my study reports weak but promising findings in a sea of otherwise strong effects, I would be much more inclined to draw optimistic conclusions. Studies never stand in isolation, and they never should. Finally, I would not be inclined to offer policy recommendations. In my view, that is the job of what Cronbach et al. (1980) called the policy-shaping community.

WHAT OTHER LESSONS CAN WE LEARN?

If we turned back the clock, the researchers might have done two things to minimize the chances that the dilemma they faced would occur. The first is a competent power analysis based on the size of an effect that would make a policy difference. If that was not done, serious ethical questions exist about the waste of resources potentially inherent in mounting such a large and presumably expensive study. The second is to ensure that this study grew out of an existing literature that strongly suggested the intervention is likely to be effective. In the latter case, meta-analysis of existing studies is increasingly being used to help design future interventions so as to take maximum advantage of past knowledge and existing resources. For example, the British journal *The Lancet* recently announced that papers submitted for publication should show that they either did or consulted a meta-analysis of previous research during the design of the study.

CONCLUSION

For me, at least, this case does not pose a difficult ethical dilemma. However, it does highlight the specialized knowledge required to ensure that the high-technical-standards component of the Systematic Inquiry principle is met. Evaluation has thankfully become a field in which multiple methodologies are the norm. It happens that I am an expert in randomized field trials, so I have sufficient experience and technical knowledge to know what details to look for. Had the evaluation in this case used an ethnography, a survey, or a management-information-system methodology, the relevant expertise I would have brought to bear would have been much more generalized and limited.

REFERENCES

American Evaluation Association. (2004). *Guiding principles for evaluators* (rev.). Available at *www.eval.org/Publications/GuidingPrinciples.asp*.

Cronbach, L. J., Ambron, S. R., Dornbusch, S. M., Hess, R. D., Hornik, R. C., Phillips, D. C., et al. (1980). *Toward reform of program evaluation*. San Francisco: Jossey-Bass.

Fisher, R. A. (1926). The arrangement of field experiments. *Journal of the Ministry of Agriculture of Great Britain, 33*, 505–513.

Joint Committee on Standards for Educational Evaluation. (1994). *The program evaluation standards: How to assess evaluations of educational programs* (2nd ed.). Thousand Oaks, CA: Sage.

Rosnow, R. L., & Rosenthal, R. (1989). Statistical procedures and the justification of knowledge in psychological science. *American Psychologist, 44*, 1276–1284.

■   ■   ■   ■

WHAT IF . . . ?

. . . the pattern of results found in this evaluation had not been generated by a "strong randomized design" but by a less powerful, quasi-experimental one?

. . . anecdotal data suggest that the conservation program suffered from implementation problems that could have weakened the potency of the intervention?

. . . the conservation program was relatively inexpensive compared with other city-wide conservation initiatives?

FINAL THOUGHTS

Knock, Knock, What's There?

An evaluator's ethical responsibility for "getting the technical stuff right" is at the core of Cooksy's and Shadish's reflections on this scenario. Whether the focus is on the methodological decisions made by the evaluator (Systematic Inquiry) or the relevant knowledge and skills possessed by the evaluation team (Competence), both commentators emphasize that there are right ways and wrong ways of analyzing the data in this situation and that the team needs to understand these differences and make the appropriate choices. Failure to do so not only violates the Systematic Inquiry and Competence principles but also threatens the principles of Integrity/Honesty, Respect for People, and Responsibilities for General and Public Welfare. Indeed, one can imagine that the situation the evaluators find themselves in results, at least in part, from methodological missteps *earlier* in the study (e.g., lack of attention to power analysis or using data of poor quality). Cooksy and Shadish further note that it is important for the team to view the results of their research within the context of other evaluations in the energy conservation domain. Taking such a meta-analytic perspective is consistent with, and would seem to be implicitly required by, the Systematic Inquiry principle.

Overall, then, Cooksy and Shadish appear to be pretty much "on the same page" in their substantive review of this case. They agree that

Jake's position is untenable and that a more sophisticated analysis of the evaluation data is called for both methodologically and ethically. And they agree on at least the general outline of what this analysis would look like. Cooksy may be more confident than Shadish that a single study can have a significant impact on policymakers' decisions, but this difference in perspective does not reflect an *ethical* disagreement. On the central ethical issues is this case, there seems to be consensus.

Things Happen

For the past 2 years, the local visiting nurses association has sponsored a program that provides a network of services to the elderly in low-income sections of the city. Less than a year ago, the association initiated a support program for the nurses who work in this intensive and demanding outreach effort. Shortly after the latter program began, you were hired to evaluate its impact on participants' self-reported beliefs, attitudes, feelings, skills, and interests. At first you were reluctant to take on the job, given that the staff overseeing the support program had already administered a pretest survey they had designed to measure these variables. This meant that you would have to work within the constraints imposed by this instrument. You decided that it *would* be possible to conduct a valid evaluation under these circumstances, and added a number of questions to the original survey that would be used in the follow-up survey at the end of the 6-month support intervention. You also planned to interview as many of the participating nurses as you could after the program ended.

After the association had accepted your proposal, you attended a few of the weekly support sessions so that you would not have to rely solely on the written program description to get a sense of the specific dimensions that the intervention was intended to affect. You found that the program in practice reflected quite closely the program as planned. In the months that followed, you were in regular contact with the support program's staff, and they consistently assured you that the intervention was running smoothly.

Fast forward to the present. The support program recently ended, and you have begun to interview participants. And all does *not* appear to be well. About halfway through the program, one of the nurses had been robbed at gunpoint during a visit to a client in a public housing project. At the time, the staff had informed you of the event but said nothing to indicate that the support program had been affected in a way that would have implications for the evaluation. It turns out, however, that in response to the robbery the support sessions increasingly began to focus on issues of safety, often to the neglect of other issues that were supposed to be covered in the "curriculum." When you review the follow-up surveys completed by participants, your fears are confirmed. On nearly all of the dimensions that the intervention was designed to address, no pre–post differences were found. Surprisingly, this was the case even for the survey items dealing with safety-related concerns. It appears, based on your interviews, that the session facilitators handled discussions of safety in a manner that did not reduce participants' sense of vulnerability.

It is unfortunate that the support program coordinator did not display more candor in describing to you the influence of the robbery on the sessions. You might have been able to modify the postprogram survey and perhaps add a midcourse survey as well to target in a more refined, responsive fashion some of the areas that the "revised" program did manage to address with at least some success. As things currently stand, the data suggest that the support intervention was pretty much of a bust, a verdict that may be excessively bleak.

The bottom line is that you want your data analysis to be fair to the program, and you're not sure that the data you have enable you to achieve that goal. However, the intuitive appeal of a support program for these nurses may be affecting your judgment. Is your belief in the inherent worth of such an intervention getting in the way of looking objectively at what actually took place over the past 6 months? You don't relish the task of data analysis and interpretation that awaits you, and you're not sure of the best way to handle it.

QUESTIONS TO CONSIDER

1. Do you bear any *ethical* responsibility for the failure to adapt the evaluation to the changing circumstances of the support program? Why or why not?

2. What are the most important differences between this case and the Knock, Knock, What's There scenario?

3. Would you mention in your written evaluation report that you were not informed of the change in the program that occurred as a result of the robbery?

4. In what ways is the challenge you face in analyzing and interpreting the data in this case an ethical challenge?

5. If the data collected about this intervention had only consisted of postprogram interviews, would this affect the ethics of the situation you're dealing with now?

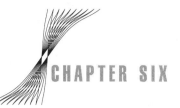

CHAPTER SIX

Communication of Results

Mainstream

In the often frustrating world of welfare-to-work programs, the 2-year-old Main-stream Academy initiative, sponsored by the Department of Employment Services in your state, has received a great deal of attention. In many such interventions, welfare recipients are quickly placed in low-wage jobs in the service sector that offer little hope of upward mobility. Mainstream's agenda is much more ambitious. It provides participants with an intensive, coordinated network of education, training, socialization, and support services for a period of up to 20 months. Those who successfully "graduate" from the academy are guaranteed a job offer from at least one of the employers that have an ongoing relationship with the program. These jobs are not dead-end; they come with salaries and medical benefits that are intended to represent a route out of poverty that is sustainable in the long term.

For the past several months, you have been conducting a process evaluation of Mainstream Academy's six sites scattered throughout the state.

Last week you submitted a draft of your findings to the Department of Employment Services, which is funding the evaluation. Your report is due to be released within the next month. The results of an impact evaluation, conducted by another evaluator, will not be available for at least another 1½ years.

You are meeting with the department's deputy director to discuss your draft, and a problem has arisen. The deputy director objects to a section of the report that describes discontent among a number of White staff members at two of the sites. These staff claim that they sometimes feel pressured by their superiors to lower performance standards for African American participants to ensure that African Americans are well represented among the academy's graduates. In this section of the draft, you also indicate that superiors at these sites maintain that they routinely encourage staff to display flexibility in working with *all* academy participants but that they do not advocate that standards be lowered. These superiors note that differences between White staff members and African American participants in their social class and cultural backgrounds can pose distinctive challenges to the former when they attempt to be appropriately, and effectively, flexible.

The deputy director would like you to delete this section of the findings. In his view, "What good can come of this? You report no hard evidence showing that performance standards have been compromised, or even that genuine pressure has been brought to bear. No formal grievances have been filed by staff. All you've got is a classic case of "We say . . . , They say . . ." with a racial angle thrown in. The last thing this program needs right now in the eyes of the public is a Black–White controversy that evokes images of reverse discrimination and God knows what else. Without solid data to back up these accusations, I think it's irresponsible to introduce such a volatile issue into the report. You'll just be pandering to a small group of malcontents who are intent on stirring up trouble."

You are not unsympathetic to the deputy director's concerns, but you have some concerns of your own. You remind him that stakeholder perceptions typically represent a key component of a comprehensive process evaluation, and that two sites out of six is not a negligible proportion. What's more, these two sites contain 40% of the program's participants. As far as the racial angle is concerned, you can't change what the staff's complaints are about; they are what they are. And although it is true that not all White staff at these two sites voiced complaints, it is also the case that *no* minority staff at these locations perceived a problem with performance standards.

Your response does little to ease the deputy director's angst, nor does it lessen his determination to remove the standards discussion from your report.

"Okay," he says, "Here's my suggestion. Let's hand over the performance standards issue to the team doing the outcome evaluation. If they find credible evidence of lower standards for African American participants, they can address the problem in detail in their report. But it wouldn't be mentioned in your report that comes out next month. Discussing this matter in print now would be premature. It's just too easy to yell "Fire" in a crowded movie theater. What do you think? Is this a reasonable compromise?"

Mainstreaming Process Evaluation: Ethical Issues in Reporting Interim Results

Mary Ann Scheirer

The case of Mainstream Academy seems, at first glance, to be a classic instance of a program executive's attempt to bury negative findings. The evaluator's early process evaluation revealed hints from several White staff members that they "are pressured" to lower performance standards for African American participants in this ambitious welfare-to-work program. The department's deputy director wants you to delete this part of your written report, while you, as a conscientious evaluator, feel that *all* the findings ought to be reported, even if they are negative. My commentary discusses the ethical issues underlying this situation and proposes alternatives to both strategies presented in the scenario: the deputy director's suggestion to ignore these findings until the outcome report comes out in 18 months, and the evaluator's belief that the staff members may be raising valid concerns that should be included in the written report. I will assume that the evaluator in this case is an external evaluator, funded by a contract with the Department of Employment Services.

DIAGNOSING THE CONTEXT: PROCESS EVALUATION IN THE EARLY STAGE

It appears that the finding in question arose from a set of interviews using qualitative methods, early in the evaluation assignment. Perhaps they were discussions with a sample of the staff members, or with all staff members in the six sites, to obtain their perceptions of the operations of Mainstream Academy and to surface additional issues that the process evaluation should include. That would be a good initial step in conducting reconnaissance about the situation, before devising a full plan for the process and outcome (impact) evaluations. So far, no other types of data have been collected that might illuminate the issue of whether the standards are the same for all participants. Rather than focus now on a written report of findings from this set of interviews, it might be preferable for the evaluator to do a more thorough job of reconnoitering the situation. Is there a logic model that clearly specifies the intended activities and services of the academy itself as well as what is expected of participants? Are there well-developed performance standards for participants? What other types of data might be routinely collected to help shed light on this situation? For example, are there attendance data? Records of other types of participation by clients? Are there interim tests or other assessments of client progress at the academy that would yield information about their performance? Diagnosing the context of the program being evaluated and learning about already-available data that might be useful in the study are key steps in process evaluation.

WHAT IS PROCESS EVALUATION AND WHY DO IT?

Further analysis of the Mainstream scenario requires an understanding of process evaluation and its role in this case. Although there can be many reasons and purposes for process evaluation (cf. Scheirer, 1994), let's assume that the major objective here is to provide data for feedback to program managers to improve the operations, and thus the outcomes, of the academy. When contracting for the process evaluation, the department wanted to know if its intended program is being implemented well in each of the six sites as well as to have the evaluator's recommendations for improvement. Thus, the report that the evaluator is being asked to change is likely to be an early report from a utilization-focused evaluation, not a major summative report. Further, I assume that there were *not* prior claims of racial bias in the program that were to be investigated by this process evaluation.

The role of an evaluator in management-focused process evaluation is often quite different from the role adopted when conducting research about program efficacy. To provide appropriate feedback, a process evaluator needs to have a good understanding of the details of the program—in this case, the academy—to know how it is operating. The evaluator needs to be *strategic* in working with program managers in terms of using a variety of communication methods, in recommending types of data to be collected, and in framing findings and suggestions for action. A process evaluator is often a coach for data-collection planning, an aide in analyzing and interpreting data collected by others, and/or a facilitator of management development processes using data.

Developing a program logic model as the first step toward process evaluation can help to assess the potential utility of different types of process data as well as to be sure there is consensus among stakeholders about intended program components and outcomes. If resources for collecting data are limited, as they usually are, strategic decisions need to be made about the types of data to be collected, who will collect it, and how feedback from the process evaluation will be provided. In this case, few of these steps in developing a working relationship with the client and developing an initial understanding of the program seem to have been accomplished. It may be premature to offer a written report on just one piece of what should have been a fuller "getting-to-know-you" stage of the process.

Given that Mainstream's intended program is an "ambitious" package, including a "coordinated network of education, training, socialization, and support services," it will be important for the process evaluation to focus on the fidelity of implementation across the six sites and over time. How can this program vision be translated into a well-defined set of program components to be delivered appropriately in sites with a diversity of participants? Are there tools in place for measuring the fidelity of its implementation, or do these tools need to be created by the process evaluation? The evaluator knows that prior evaluations of such complex interventions have shown that their ambitions often exceed their grasp, and the actual programs as delivered do not implement all the components. So it will be essential to measure fidelity of implementation rigorously, in order to help increase it, if needed, and to connect that data to the data being collected by the impact evaluator.

But let's assume that the contracted process evaluation included only a set of interviews and requires a written report for this short time period. You are faced with a decision about whether to delete (or change) the offending sections, to insist that those sections be retained as written, or to find a compromise solution that still allows you to ethically perform the role of a process evaluator. What to *do*?

WHAT EVALUATION GUIDING PRINCIPLES APPLY HERE?

The ethical evaluator might suggest to the deputy director that they jointly consult the Guiding Principles for Evaluators. Doing this would give you and the deputy director time to consider the various ethical principles involved and avoid increasing any tension that has arisen between the two of you. You both agree to study the Guiding Principles, consider further alternatives, and meet again next week. You find that all of the following principles have some relevance in this situation:

• *Integrity/Honesty*: "[Evaluators] represent accurately their procedures, data, and findings, and attempt to prevent or correct misuse of their work by others" (American Evaluation Association, 2004, Principle C-5); *Responsibilities for General and Public Welfare*: "[Evaluators] include relevant perspectives and interests of the full range of stakeholders" (Principle E-1). You are concerned that simply deleting the finding that some staff members feel they are pressured to use different standards for members of different racial groups would violate the principle of accurately presenting your findings from this initial set of interviews. Further, if some staff members believed this perception was important enough to report, would you be denying them a proper voice as program stakeholders if you delete their perspectives? And, perhaps more important to the process evaluation, if the allegations are correct and some participants are not meeting the same standards as others during their participation in the program, would these individuals be able to pass final examinations for graduation from the program or for certification needed for employment? Waiting another 18 months for the results from an impact evaluation is a long time to let this issue simmer and fester, if it is indeed a valid issue.

• *Systematic Inquiry*: "[Evaluators] adhere to the highest technical standards appropriate to the methods they use" (American Evaluation Association, 2004, Principle A-1). You realize that the interviews conducted thus far represent only one of several methods that could be used in this process evaluation. Drawing findings from multiple methods to confirm politically sensitive conclusions would apply higher technical standards than using any single data source. The deputy director's concern about the absence of "hard evidence" for this finding suggests the need for more than one source of data. Further, in your haste to get started on the project, you acknowledge that you interviewed those staff members who were available and willing to be interviewed during your 1-day visit to each site rather than interviewing a systematically chosen, representative sample of staff. The claims of lower performance standards for some participants may just be "sour grapes" from a few staff members who are disgruntled for other reasons. The "highest technical standards" for this politically volatile issue would seem to call for further data collection.

• *Competence*: "[Evaluators] ensure that the evaluation team collectively demonstrates cultural competence" (American Evaluation Association, 2004, Principle B-2). Issues of cultural competence might be important to explore here both among the staff members at the local sites and yourself as an evaluator. Were you, as a White, Anglo evaluator, too ready to accept on face value these claims of reverse racial bias from White staff members? In your interviews, did you adequately explore what those interviewees meant by "feeling pressured . . . to lower performance standards for African American participants"? Given that these concerns were voiced, is there a need for further staff training on how to overcome potential barriers in communication among staff and participants of diverse backgrounds?

• *Respect for People*: "[Evaluators] seek a comprehensive understanding of the contextual elements of the evaluation" (American Evaluation Association, 2004, Principle D-1). As indicated previously, you realize that you have not yet done the reconnaissance needed to understand the full situation here. Your work thus far has not included understanding the standards being used for participants in the program and how they are currently assessed. Further, you may not be aware of racial tensions that have been going on for some time and any efforts already made to diffuse them.

• *Respect for People*: "[Evaluators] seek to maximize the benefits and reduce any unnecessary harms that might occur from an evaluation and carefully judge when the benefits from the evaluation or procedure should be forgone because of potential risks" (American Evaluation Association, 2004, Principle D-3); *Responsibilities for General and Public Welfare*: "Consider not only immediate operations and outcomes of the evaluation, but also the broad assumptions, implications and potential side effects" (Principle E-2). These principles seem very relevant here: Formal reporting of a preliminary and perhaps rather minor point in a broader initial report might increase racial tensions rather than diffuse them. Moreover, insisting on keeping this point in a formal report might jeopardize the relationship of trust in evaluation that you are trying to build with the deputy director and the department. You want them to invest in a more comprehensive process evaluation system that will provide adequate feedback on the fidelity of implementing program components. Perhaps this first set of interviews provides hints that many intended components of the full academy program have questionable local implementation. It could be essential to achieving intended participant outcomes that program managers put in place a systematic process evaluation to provide timely feedback on the entire program.

This examination of the Guiding Principles reveals that they are relevant to the Mainstream scenario, but they do not provide uniform guidance. The principles call for accurately reporting findings and for including the voices of all stakeholders, yet also emphasize making sure your technical procedures are strong enough and considering carefully the potential consequences of your actions as an evaluator. Conflicting guidance from multiple principles often occurs in the messy, real world of evaluation practice. Morris (2005) suggests an ethical cost–benefit analysis to help resolve these conflicts by comparing "the ethical risks of an evaluation with the social good that the evaluation is likely to produce" (p. 133). In the Mainstream case, the benefits of retaining in the formal written report the contested section emerging from the early stage of the process evaluation are likely to be much lower than the potential costs to the program of increased racial tension or of failing to continue the process evaluation long enough to assess full implementation of this complex program. Given that the key purpose of process evaluation here is to provide early feedback about the status and fidelity of implementation, you have *already* provided some feedback by raising the standards issue in a draft report. Further actions to follow up on this potential problem are desirable, without necessarily including the issue with this wording in a formal written report. In addition, it is very undesirable to have a tug of war on this issue with the deputy director. Several other action strategies are possible rather than simply waiting for another 18 months or so until the impact evaluation is available.

POTENTIAL SOLUTIONS

A first step would be to suggest to the deputy director that this issue be examined within the broader process evaluation that you are still designing. An important question to explore in this regard is, What are the "standards" that some staff members believe are not being upheld? What did they mean by this comment, and how could the standards be examined *systematically*? The very first Guiding Principle states that "evaluators conduct systematic, data-based inquiries" (American Evaluation Association, 2004, Principle A). The future process evaluation could examine the accuracy and reliability of data collected for these standards or establish new data-collection methods for them if none currently exist. This could be done in the context of developing (or making more systematic) a data system to track the fidelity of Mainstream's program implementation across the six sites, including

its standards for participants. For example, are data about participants' attendance and participation being collected and examined frequently? Such data could be used to counsel participants with frequent
absences or tardiness to help determine the reasons for their problems
and devise potential solutions. Are participants' assignments being
graded unreliably? That might call for training of staff members to cali-
brate their grading procedures.

However, your further investigation may suggest that this is a situation in which variation in participants' interaction with staff members is potentially desirable in terms of adapting the program to varying needs. For example, African American participants may be more
likely than Whites to have problems making consistent child care
arrangements, if they live in urban areas where high-quality child care
centers are full. Or if the standards issue does not refer to measurable
program components, it may suggest a need for interventions to
increase the cultural competence of staff members or for methods to
increase dialogue and communication between staff members of different races working within the same center.

Further, the major findings from this draft report should not just
be reported to the deputy director but should be the basis for verbal
feedback and discussion among all the sites. A good compromise
would be to suggest that all of the findings and recommendations from
your draft report be discussed in the next quarterly meeting of site
directors, with potential for follow-up in an "all-staff" retreat in the
summer. Issues concerning performance standards for participants in
the program, and whether they are assessed fairly for all, can be raised
without even mentioning the "racial angle." This also might be a good
opportunity for interactive training on cultural competence, perhaps
for staff members of all races to learn how to better address the needs
of participants. In this situation, changing the communication method,
from a written report to discussing the underlying issues among the
staff members involved, is likely to be much more effective in addressing these concerns.

In summary, the key issues for future process evaluation are to (1)
define the data to be collected to assess the fidelity of program implementation, including performance standards for participants (or to
reconsider them if they already exist); (2) assess the reliability and
accuracy of procedures for collecting data about performance standards; and then (3) use that data for objective feedback to staff members at least once per year and more often if feasible. The data-
feedback techniques could analyze aggregate data about participants'

scores on the standards using several demographic variables in addition to race (e.g., gender, age, rural/urban residence, level of education) to see whether all types of participants are making adequate progress in the program. This would allow examination of the potential for racial bias without raising undue alarms that might simply exacerbate racial tensions.

The evaluator should review the communication style used in the draft report just submitted. It should have a balanced and nuanced tone that reflects the report's status as an initial "cut" at examining the various components of this complex program. How was the standards finding presented in the context of other findings about the program? Was it placed among a broader set of results, or was it perhaps given undue weight because of the racial angle? Would it be acceptable to the deputy director to mention in the written report that some of those interviewed were uncertain about the application of standards for participants' achievements in the program without the additional accusation that the standards are used in a biased way? This would highlight the need to develop or assess the application of performance standards without a racial angle being raised prematurely.

Finally, it is perhaps unfortunate that the department separated "process evaluation" from "impact evaluation" in two different contracts, because these types of evaluation should be complementary and linked components of an overall evaluation strategy. Even if the impact evaluation *is* focused on establishing the efficacy of the Mainstream Academy via a rigorous comparative design, the impact evaluators will need access to process data in order to take into account, as mediating variables, the fidelity of implementation and the "dose" of program activities received by participants. For example, do participants attending a site with a fully implemented program have better outcomes than those at sites with lower fidelity to the intended program? Do participants with better attendance or higher levels of other participation variables (e.g., more homework completed or more independent practice on computers) show better outcomes than participants with a lower "dosage" of the program? Reciprocally, data about outcomes for the first cohort of participants in the impact evaluation should be examined and used for program improvement if feasible. (For example, are promises of postprogram employment kept?) This would make the use of outcome information a component of the academy's program, but this is an appropriate role for evaluation in many circumstances. Although ensuring the credibility of impact data may require that they be independently collected or verified, the outcome *findings* are not likely to be biased by sharing them at appropriate intervals with program managers. At an overall level, then, it would seem desirable to bring the two evaluation contractors together to share interim findings and avoid duplication of efforts.

Thus, a summary of steps to resolve the Mainstream case might be the following:

1. The evaluator agrees to delete this section of the interim report or to modify it by removing the racial angle while retaining some discussion of staff members' uncertainty about performance standards for participants.

2. The deputy director agrees to convene one or more meetings at which the evaluator's preliminary interview findings will be described and discussed, including a discussion of the current status of performance standards for participants and how to ensure that they are assessed accurately and fairly.

3. The evaluator will engage in a more thorough reconnoitering of the situation to learn about the background of the program, including the history of any racial tensions involved, to explore whether other types of data about the performance standards are available, and to work with program staff in developing a logic model that includes an explicit description of these standards.

4. The deputy director agrees to support the development and funding of a more comprehensive process evaluation, particularly to assess and enhance the full implementation of all program components. Further, the deputy director will convene a joint meeting of the process evaluation and impact evaluation contractors, including other relevant program stakeholders, to plan for appropriate division of labor pertaining to types of data collected, appropriate sharing of data, and timely feedback of results.

CONCLUSIONS

The Mainstream scenario illustrates the frequent interconnections of potential ethical problems with inadequate evaluation procedures. In this instance, more thorough planning of the process evaluation and more thoughtful presentation of a potentially controversial finding might have prevented the conflict. This case highlights the importance of using multiple types of data in evaluation (e.g., not just interviews), especially when the findings are likely to be controversial. Also, the major purpose of process evaluation here—providing feedback for program improvement—should affect the methods used for communicating with program managers. Formal written reports are often not the most effective way to draw attention to provocative findings, if the goal is to stimulate action steps to strengthen the program.

Of course, different conclusions about the application of ethical principles might be warranted if the evaluation situation differed. For example, if the program manager had requested deleting a major finding from an impact evaluation of the Mainstream Academy, then removing those results from a report to stakeholders would likely be a major ethical violation. Consider a situation in which an impact evaluation found major differences (both statistically and substantively significant) in both participant attendance and graduation rates, showing lower performance for African Americans than for other ethnicities. Multivariate analysis confirmed a strong relationship between attendance and the probability of graduation, with statistical controls taking into account other likely influences on the outcome variable of graduation. Assume further that evaluators had reported, at several points during the 2-year process evaluation, the problems revealed by data indicating lower attendance for some participants. However, program managers had done little to diagnose the sources of those problems or to intervene to increase attendance. In this scenario, it would be important to report the findings to political-level stakeholders, such as the state legislature, even though the findings suggest a potential weakness of program management. Why did the managers not use the data about low attendance as feedback in an attempt to improve attendance, drawing from many prior studies that show strong relationships between dosage variables, such as attendance, and intended program outcomes? In this situation, deleting the findings showing racial differences would be a serious ethical violation for both the evaluator and the program manager.

Ethical evaluation practice requires flexibility and a judgmental balance among multiple ethical principles and several courses of action. Truthful presentation of findings *is* important, but so are other principles embodied in the Guiding Principles. Assessing the potential costs and benefits of various approaches can help evaluators and program managers weigh the importance of competing ethical principles in order to create solutions acceptable to all concerned. Evaluations conducted at different stages of a program, for different purposes, may call for different applications of the American Evaluation Association's Guiding Principles. A broader consideration of ethical issues, guidelines, and possible decisions can lead to better, more useful evaluation practice.

REFERENCES

American Evaluation Association. (2004). *Guiding principles for evaluators* (rev.). Available at *www.eval.org/Publications/GuidingPrinciples.asp.*

Morris, M. (2005). Ethics. In S. Mathison (Ed.), *Encyclopedia of evaluation* (pp. 131–134). Thousand Oaks, CA: Sage.

Scheirer, M. A. (1994). Designing and using process evaluation. In J. S. Wholey, H. P. Hatry, & K. E. Newcomer (Eds.), *Handbook of practical program evaluation* (pp. 40–68). San Francisco: Jossey-Bass.

COMMENTARY

Reporting Bad News: Challenges and Opportunities in an Ethical Dilemma

Yolanda Suarez-Balcazar and Lucia Orellana-Damacela

The ethical predicament described in the Mainstream case would certainly elicit a reflective pause in any evaluator. The most urgent question, of course, is, "What do I do now?" However, our evaluator would also benefit from asking herself a second question: "How did I end up in this mess?"

Ethical issues are an essential part of evaluation (LaPolt, 1997; Turner, 2003), and high standards for ethical practice have been developed by the American Evaluation Association (2004). According to LaPolt (1997), evaluators of social programs must be prepared for ethical dilemmas at every stage of their work. The present case places the evaluator in a situation in which she has to address a common challenge: the overt pressure to avoid bad news in an evaluation report.

We have organized this commentary into two sections. In the first, we highlight some general issues that, in our opinion, help to clarify the dilemma and its potential resolution. In this regard, we discuss the evaluator's role and responsibilities, with an emphasis on the Guiding Principles for Evaluators. Another issue relevant to this case is the difference between process and outcome evaluation. The former, which explores how a program operates, is more likely to embrace "soft" data (perceptions and opinions), whereas the second, by focusing on the products of the process, emphasizes data that are usually perceived as "hard" or "tangible." This distinction is not, of course, written in stone, and any good evaluation combines both types of data. However, some evaluation consumers tend to assign higher weight or credibility to information coming from what they perceive as objective, or factual, data as opposed to subjective data. In the Mainstream scenario, that might be a reason for the deputy director's reaction.

In the second section, we explore the ethical implications of the alternative courses of action available to our beleaguered evaluator. We also retrospectively examine the decisions and actions that might have contributed to this standoff between the evaluator and the deputy director. Using the benefits of hindsight, we propose a strategy that might have helped to avoid, or at least ameliorate, the difficulties that the evaluator finds herself facing now.

THE IMPORTANCE OF CONTEXT

What Is the Responsibility of the Evaluator?

The Guiding Principle of Integrity/Honesty mandates, among other things, that evaluators "not misrepresent their procedures, data or findings [and] they should attempt to prevent or correct misuse of their work by others" (American Evaluation Association, 2004, Principle C-5). This implies not just making the "easy" ethical choices between right and wrong, but working through more complex decisions that involve hierarchies of values, prioritized according to circumstances, and deciding what is, and is not, valid and credible information (Mabry, 2004). In this case, the disagreement between the evaluator and the deputy director lies at the heart of the ethical dilemma faced by the evaluator. Should she try to persuade her client that the staff's comments should be kept in the process report, or should she agree to delete them and see what happens with the outcome evaluation? In part, the challenge is magnified by the nature of the concerns raised by the staff at two of the sites, as they relate to sensitive racial matters.

The evaluator needs to respond to the request of her client, but she has to do so without jeopardizing the interests of other stakeholders involved in the evaluation and/or affected by the results. She has an obligation to the staff members who expressed their concerns in a confidential manner, hoping that the evaluator would communicate them to upper management. If she does not include these concerns in her report, the evaluator will be ignoring their views. This may negatively impact the participation of these staff in future evaluation efforts, because they may believe that their perspectives are not taken seriously. Indeed, they might even feel deceived by the evaluator. Deception in evaluation practice, as noted by Guba and Lincoln (1988), is unethical and counterproductive.

Because of the sensitivity of racial issues, the staff might not feel comfortable bringing their complaints directly to their supervisor or the deputy director. The evaluator is serving as their "voice" and needs to find ways to communicate such information to stakeholders with decision-making power. However, even if the evaluator decides to keep the bad news in her report, the deputy director might choose not to share the report with the stakeholders or to disseminate only selected excerpts. Against this background, it should be stressed that it is the responsibility of the evaluator to try to persuade the deputy director to keep the concerns of the staff in the report.

If the evaluator decides to wait and see what happens with the outcome evaluation, at least two scenarios are possible. One is that the outcome evaluation, scheduled to be completed 18 months later, does not find hard data to support the staff's claim. The second is that the performance standards for African Americans are, in fact, discovered to be lower. In the former case, the outcome report will probably not include the concerns raised by staff in the process evaluation. The implications of the latter possibility are discussed later in this commentary.

What Is the "Truth" in This Case?

Some staff may believe that performance standards are being lowered for African Americans, but the facts may or may not support such a claim. One might ask, What is the face validity of the concern raised by the staff? Is it a perception objective enough to reflect the truth? Perhaps not: A perception, after all, is a "subjective appraisal." Nevertheless, for those staff, that perception is the truth as they see it. Their belief might be regarded by others as isolated perceptions or even office gossip that does not have strong supporting evidence. It is the job of the evaluator to make sense of all this. Gabor and Grinnell (1994), in their discussion of myths about evaluation in human services, argue that, although the words *data* and *information* are used interchangeably, the former "signifies isolated facts in numerical or descriptive form," whereas the latter is the "interpretation given to the data when they have all been collected, collated and analyzed" (p. 5). Given these definitions, the Mainstream Academy evaluator does not appear to have enough data, collected from different sources, such as clients or program records, to accurately interpret the assertions of the disgruntled staff.

On the other hand, one could argue that evaluators have a responsibility to communicate the "truth as evaluation participants see it," which, in this case, includes the concerns shared by certain staff from two of the program sites. Thus, the evaluator is not only responsible to the stakeholder who hired her (probably the deputy director) but also to participants who provide valuable evaluation-relevant information. If reporting the "whole truth" is what evaluators must strive for, then part of the truth is the issue raised by this subgroup of staff.

As noted, however, the evaluator ultimately needs to determine whether she has adequate information and process data to lend credence to the claim of these staff. As Mabry (2004) asserts, "Insufficient data may yield unintentionally skewed descriptions of program resources, contexts, process, and outcomes" (p. 387). Is the information the evaluator has sufficient? Is it credible? Is more information needed before making a decision to include or not include the perceptions of the staff members who feel that the performance standards have been lowered?

Process versus Outcome Evaluation

A central issue in this case is the significance assigned to program process. The deputy director appears to be downplaying the credibility of certain information gathered during the process evaluation. There are at least two reasons why this might be happening. The first is that he does not consider the finding in question to be sufficiently conclusive or important. An overemphasis on program outcomes can sometimes lead to the dismissing of more nuanced, richer, or deeper analyses of process, particularly when the latter analyses reveal negative dynamics.

Process evaluation, however, can provide very valuable information to new programs. It is designed to collect data about the delivery of services to populations in need and to determine the nature of those services (Gottfredson, Fink, Skroban, & Gottfredson, 1997; Miller & Cassel, 2000). Key questions that the process evaluation might address in the Mainstream Academy program are as follows: What are the characteristics of the clients? Are they a homogeneous group, or are there important differences among them that might influence how they use the program? Are the instructors appropriately trained? Have the program designer and implementers developed a model or theory of how and why the program is supposed to work?

Process evaluation is an important step that precedes outcome evaluation, because it helps clarify anticipated outcome goals, inform ways in which programs can be modified or improved, and ensure that the needs of the target population are met (Suarez-Balcazar & Harper, 2003). In addition, process evaluation can yield information about implementation that might or might not be corroborated by the outcome evaluation (Linney & Wandersman, 1996). Thus, this evaluation has a rightful place in an evaluation effort, generating key findings that might not otherwise be revealed in an outcome study. In the Mainstream case, the perceptions of program staff are likely to hold great value for shaping the program.

A second reason for the deputy director's refusal to accept the findings is that he might dispute the methodological credibility of the information. If the evaluation relied exclusively on interviews with staff, without proper triangulation or corroboration from other sources (such as organizational records), then the issue of lower performance standards should not be included in the report as a *finding* but rather as a *question* to be further explored.

WHAT SHOULD THE EVALUATOR DO NOW?

To answer this question, the evaluator must weigh the pros and cons of the alternatives. For the purposes of this discussion, we will assume that she believes that the concerns raised by staff are offered in good faith and not born out of a desire to harm the program. We also assume that the evaluator does not consider the statements about unequal application of performance standards a "proven fact"; rather, they represent a starting point for a more comprehensive inquiry into the matter.

Going Along with the Deputy Director

To maintain a good working relationship with the deputy director, the evaluator might choose to go along with his suggestion and remove the bad news from the current report and wait until the outcome evaluation report is ready. She may decide to take this course of action to avoid a confrontation with the deputy director or because she believes the claim made by the staff needs to be substantiated with hard outcome data.

At first glance, this solution seems reasonable. However, we believe that it depends on too many "ifs." It assumes that the deputy director will be around to inform the outcome evaluation team of the need to examine the issue in question *and* that he will, in fact, communicate the issue to them. When the outcome report is submitted, the evaluation could yield hard data supporting the staff's concerns, or it could not. In the former case, going along with the deputy director assumes that he will not attempt to bury that outcome. Such openness would represent a departure from his previous behavior, when he tried to remove sensitive material from the process report. Indeed, nothing guarantees that the same response will not occur at the summative evaluation phase.

In short, by selecting the going-along alternative, the evaluator remains on good terms with the deputy director, but there is no assurance that the controversial question raised by the staff will be addressed. The ethical soundness of this strategy would be strengthened if the evaluator became actively involved in ensuring that the outcome evaluation team learned about the staff's complaints and encouraged the team to include the issue of performance standards in their evaluation plan.

Going against the Deputy Director

The evaluator, of course, could resist the pressure from the deputy director and keep the comments from the staff in her report. By doing so, she might harm her relationship with him, and the deputy director could choose to terminate her services sooner rather than later.

In this regard, it is important to note that the Guiding Principle of Respect for People states that evaluators should seek a "comprehensive understanding of the important contextual elements of the evaluation" (American Evaluation Association, 2004, Principle D-1), such as the political and social climates. In other words, evaluators should not provide unsubstantiated ammunition to program detractors, which is what the deputy director suspects will happen if the section of the report in dispute is included. Evaluators are also advised by the same principle to "maximize the benefits and reduce any unnecessary harm" to participants and "not compromise the integrity of the evaluation findings" (Principle D-3).

With these considerations in mind, our evaluator could try to ameliorate the controversy and improve the likelihood of the information being disseminated by managing *how* it is reported. According to Fawcett et al. (1996), communicating results is a critical aspect of evaluation because findings represent potential tools for social change and action. As in this case, conflicts are likely to arise when deciding what to report and how to report it (Posavac & Carey, 2003). If the evaluator chooses to include the comments made by some of the program staff about the performance standards being lowered, she should carefully consider how to report this perception to minimize the chances of the information being deleted or ignored. Typical ways of doing this include presenting first the "good news" about the program (e.g., employing positive quotes from participants and staff) and raising the issue of performance standards in a section entitled, for example, "Areas in Need of Improvement According to Program Staff."

It is possible that the evaluator can bring the deputy director on board if she reports the statements about standards as compelling evaluation *questions* that need to be further explored. This would focus attention on the possibility of inconsistent or uneven application of standards without emphasizing the racial aspect of the issue. She should stress the fact that she is also giving voice to the site managers' view that they encourage flexibility in working with *all* participants, without advocating any lowering of standards.

The evaluator could clarify that these perceptions of program staff need to be substantiated when the outcome evaluation report is published. Alternatively, depending on what was previously agreed on regarding the scope of the evaluation, the evaluator might, within the framework of her process evaluation, request an extension to collect the additional information deemed necessary to elucidate the issue.

The premise of this course of action is that the evaluator can convince the deputy director to agree to the reporting of the performance standards issue based on how she communicates it. She would state the need to examine the information in light of what additional data collection might reveal. The evaluator would be walking a tightrope between not being dismissive of the complaint and not accepting it uncritically. There is no conclusive evidence, but the recurring statements call for a thorough review.

Although this alternative is more ethically sound than the previous one, it might not work. The deputy director could refuse to go along with it, even if he is assured that differing performance standards will not be presented as a fact. Moreover, this course of action leaves out a part of the evaluator's role that is crucial in process evaluation: facilitating insight and learning.

A Third Approach?: Evaluator as Facilitator

Clearly, the discussion of the final report is not the timeliest moment in an evaluation process to start promoting organizational learning. However, in this scenario, the evaluator believes that the statements made by the staff regarding unfair application of performance standards deserve serious attention. The evaluator's goal is to convince the deputy director to include them in the report, because she believes that is the best way to ensure they will be further investigated. She is also ready to acknowledge that such statements are not facts and is willing to make that explicit in the report. However, she recognizes that perceptions shared by a significant number of staff members create the sense of reality under which these members operate, regardless of the dynamics they spring from within the organization. As such, these socially created realities have an impact on the program's day-to-day operations and, quite possibly, its outcomes.

Thus, the evaluator wants not only to persuade the deputy director of the importance of reporting the information in question but to change his mind-set toward the issue. She wants to show him that learning and organizational improvement can occur by embracing the issue rather than avoiding it. Granted, this goal would be easier to achieve if a climate of trust and open discussion had been established from the beginning of the process.

The evaluator might begin by telling the deputy director that the fact that these employees have expressed their complaints is a *positive* sign that they trust something can be done within the organization to address the issue. However, if their complaints do not find their rightful place in the report, they might feel alienated and betrayed and could even go outside the program to air their concerns. This would increase the likelihood of a public controversy focused on the fairness with which the performance standards are applied. From this perspective, it is in the best interest of the organization to give voice and respectful consideration to the expressions of these staff members in a precisely worded formal report.

Furthermore, the evaluator might suggest forming a work group that includes the process and outcome evaluators and representatives of all the main stakeholders (the deputy director as well as staff members, supervisors, and participants from the different sites). This group would discuss the issue and determine what information needs to be gathered regarding application of the standards. Data collection and analysis can be done by the outcome evaluator, by the process evaluator, or by both working together. The evaluator should emphasize that a finding that the standards have been lowered for a particular group would provide an opportunity for program improvement.

The key question would then become, "If this is happening, what are the reasons?" Is it due to deficiencies in the training of the staff? Is it because the program is addressing more effectively the needs of some groups than others? Which particular areas of the program are not responding to the needs of specific groups? Thus, it is important that the evaluators look beyond race to discover why some groups are less able than others to take full advantage of the program. Is it lower educational levels when they enter the program? Health problems? Lack of social support? Single parenthood?

The evaluator should consider engaging in an in-depth discussion of these issues with the deputy director. African Americans are more likely than other clients to come into the human services system with severe limitations and challenges. This is not surprising, given that they often grow up in environments characterized by limited opportunities and histories of segregation, oppression, and discrimination (Belgrave, 1998; Jencks, 1993; Wheaton, Finch, Wilson, & Granello, 1997). The program may need to take these environments into account in the design of performance standards to accommodate participant needs. The evaluator can play a role in assisting the deputy director in thinking through and investigating these matters. Indeed, if the outcome evaluation shows that the program is producing the expected outcomes, and the application of flexible standards has contributed to such success, then a systematized and explicit degree of flexibility in the application of standards by staff should be included in program training and implementation.

Ultimately, the Guiding Principle of Integrity/Honesty, which states that the evaluator should not misrepresent data or findings, demands that the Mainstream Academy evaluator keep the issue of performance standards in the report *in some form*. She should refuse to sign a report that does not include it. Otherwise, she will betray the trust of those staff who came forward and deprive the program of the chance to explore ways to improve the program's service to participants.

Decreasing the Likelihood of Ethical Dilemmas

Even with an impressive array of skills in methodology, facilitation, and consensus building, evaluators can find themselves in ethical "messes." However, there are steps one can take to decrease the likelihood of such conflicts, including the one that occurred in the Mainstream case. The evaluator could start with an explicit evaluation contract that specifies the evaluation plan and stipulates the decision-making strategies that will be followed in terms of what will be included in the process evaluation, how the evaluation will be used, and how it will provide input to the outcome evaluation.

A recommended technique is to envision different result scenarios and examine how different parties might react to them (Posavac &

Carey, 2003). Also, as a part of the contract, one should include how, when, and with whom the results will be shared. As the Guiding Principle of Responsibilities for General and Public Welfare states, evaluators "have a special relationship with the client who funds or requests the evaluation" (American Evaluation Association, 2004, Principle E-4). The client, in this case, appears to be the deputy director. The same principle indicates that evaluators "should include relevant perspectives and interests of the full range of stakeholders" and "have obligations that encompass the public interest and good" (Principles E-1 and E-5). As we understand these principles, our evaluator cannot afford to be blinded by her relationship with her client, omit relevant perspectives, and still honor the public good as the overall justification for her evaluative endeavor.

The best way for the evaluator to ensure that all relevant perspectives are included is to solicit participation from a wide array of stakeholders, including the deputy director, staff, supervisors and participants from the multiple sites, representatives from agencies that provide training or other services to participants, and representatives from the program's funder, the Department of Employment Services. In this way the information collected and analyzed will encompass multiple perspectives. The final report will not come as a surprise to anyone, and the power of any given stakeholder to manipulate or omit information will be minimized. As the evaluation is planned and its findings are discussed, new learning about the program will occur, and a shared perception of what the program is, how it works, and what it produces will be created or refined.

This process will help generate an overall vision of what the program *should* accomplish and how those accomplishments *should* be pursued. By making the discussion of the evaluation findings and their meaning a collaborative effort, the evaluator greatly reduces the possibility that one person (in this case, the deputy director) can hijack the process and shape the presentation of results to conform to his or her own agenda, values, and interest.

REFERENCES

American Evaluation Association. (2004). *Guiding principles for evaluators* (rev.). Available at *www.eval.org/Publications/GuidingPrinciples.asp.*

Belgrave, F. Z. (1998). *Psychosocial aspects of chronic illness and disability among African Americans.* Richmond, VA: Virginia Commonwealth University.

Fawcett, S. B., Paine-Andrews, A., Francisco, V. T., Schultz, J. A., Ritcher, K. P., Lewis, R. K., et al. (1996). Empowering community health initiatives through evaluation. In D. M. Fetterman, S. Kaftarian, & A. Wandersman (Eds.), *Empowerment evaluation: Knowledge and tools for self-assessment and accountability* (pp. 161–187). Thousand Oaks, CA: Sage.

Gabor P., & Grinnell R., Jr. (1994). *Evaluation and quality improvement in the human services.* Boston: Allyn & Bacon.

Gottfredson, D. C., Fink, C. M., Skroban, S., & Gottfredson, G. D. (1997). Making prevention work. In R. P. Weissberg, T. P. Gullotta, R. L. Hampton, B. A. Ryan, & G. R. Adams (Eds.), *Issues in children's and families' lives: Vol. 9. Healthy children 2010—Establishing preventive services* (pp. 219–252). Thousand Oaks, CA: Sage.

Guba, E. G., & Lincoln, Y. (1988). Do inquiry paradigms imply inquiry methodologies? In D. M. Fetterman (Ed.), *Qualitative approaches to evaluation in education* (pp. 89–115). New York: Praeger.

Jencks, C. (1993). *Rethinking social policy: Race, poverty, and the underclass.* Cambridge, MA: Harvard University Press.

LaPolt, E. K. (1997). *Ethical dilemmas in program evaluation and research design.* Retrieved February 28, 2006, from *www.socialresearchmethods.net/tutorial/Lapolt/lizhtm.htm.*

Linney, J., & Wandersman, A. (1996). Empowering community groups with evaluation skills: The prevention plus III model. In D. M. Fetterman, S. J. Kaftarian, & A. Wandersman (Eds.), *Empowerment evaluation: Knowledge and tools for self-assessment and accountability* (pp. 259–276). Thousand Oaks, CA: Sage.

Mabry, L. (2004). Commentary: "Gray skies are gonna clear up." *American Journal of Evaluation, 25,* 385–390.

Miller, R. L., & Cassel, J. B. (2000). Ongoing evaluation in AIDS–service organizations: Building meaningful evaluation activities. *Journal of Prevention and Intervention in the Community, 19*(1), 21–40.

Posavac, E., & Carey, R. (2003). *Program evaluation: Methods and case studies* (6th ed.). Upper Saddle River, NJ: Prentice Hall.

Suarez-Balcazar, Y., & Harper, G. (2003). *Empowerment and participatory evaluation of community interventions: Multiple benefits.* New York: Haworth Press.

Turner, D. (2003). *Evaluation ethics and quality: Results of a survey of Australasian Evaluation Society members.* Retrieved March 6, 2006, from *www.aes.asn.au/about/ethics_survey_ summary.pdf.*

Wheaton, J. E., Finch, J., Wilson, K. B., & Granello, D. (1997). Patterns of services to vocational rehabilitation consumers based upon sex, race, and closure status. *Journal of Rehabilitation Administration, 20,* 209–225.

WHAT IF . . . ?

*. . . you did, in fact, find supporting evidence for the staff members'
accusations, and still the deputy director pleads with you not to raise
the issue in your written report? The deputy director argues that the
most effective way to address the performance standards problem is
"under the radar" and that he needs time to do that. He's afraid that
putting the issue into the report could cause the problem to "explode"
in a public fashion, fueling the conflict in a way that would make it
extremely difficult, if not impossible, to resolve constructively.*

*. . . there was no impact evaluator to hand over the performance
standards issue to?*

*. . . you failed to find solid evidence of compromised performance
standards (despite a thorough search for it), but the aggrieved staff
remain adamant that the issue is a valid one that should be raised in
your written report?*

FINAL THOUGHTS

Mainstream

As indicated in Chapter One, pressure from a stakeholder to alter the
presentation of findings is one of the most frequent—and vexing—
ethical problems encountered by evaluators. Such a challenge is at the
heart of the Mainstream scenario. Of course, this challenge might not
have occurred if the evaluator had investigated more thoroughly the
original claim made by the staff members in question.

The responses of our commentators to this dilemma are similar
but not identical. Suarez-Balcazar and Orellana-Damacela conclude
that the performance standards issue must be included in the written
report *"in some form."* Scheirer does not insist that the formal report reference the matter, but she does believe that, at a general level, the topic
of performance standards needs to be put on the table for discussion as
the evaluation unfolds.

Both Scheirer and Suarez-Balcazar and Orellana-Damacela encourage the evaluator to consider downplaying the racial angle of this

finding for the time being; they note that racial issues are inherently volatile and that the data collected thus far do not provide sufficient evidence to support a claim of bias. Introducing race into the conversation is almost certain to increase tension, and reducing that tension is likely to be a difficult task no matter how well managed the process is. Situations in which it makes sense for an evaluator to deliberately escalate conflict among stakeholders are rare.

The commentators' analyses remind us that deciding *how* to present findings can be just as crucial as deciding on *what* findings to present. This is particularly true when the *what* is controversial, a circumstance that frequently raises the ethical stakes involved. In the case of Mainstream Academy, both Scheirer and Suarez-Balcazar and Orellana-Damacela recommend a process that brings key stakeholders together to explore the performance standards issue in a positive, collaborative, problem-solving environment. In a related vein, the commentators also share a desire to link the process and outcome evaluations in a more meaningful fashion than has apparently occurred thus far.

Would you insist on raising the performance standards issue in the written report if you were the evaluator in this case? How much data does an evaluator need before he or she can ethically justify bringing a problem to the attention of stakeholders? Judgment calls such as these can be much easier to make in theory than in practice, especially when the decisions require prioritizing among various ethical principles (e.g., Systematic Inquiry and Honesty/Integrity).

Moreover, decisions to minimize conflict carry risks of their own. Omitting the racial angle from your written or verbal report *now* might lead to accusations of suppression or censorship *later* if racial bias does eventually emerge as a topic for discussion. The power of such allegations, even when they are unfounded, to taint and cripple an evaluation should never be underestimated. Evaluators must be concerned with the *appearance* of impropriety as much as they are with the *substance* of impropriety. As the Mainstream case shows, this can be a considerable burden for an evaluator to shoulder.

Whose Voices?

As the associate director of evaluation at a philanthropic foundation, you have recently concluded an evaluation of Community Voices, an initiative sponsored by the foundation in three small cities in the state. The centerpiece of Community Voices was a series of community forums facilitated by external consultants hired by the foundation. These meetings brought together local residents, elected officials, and representatives from public agencies, private agencies, and community groups throughout the city to discuss the challenges and opportunities associated with the high levels of immigration into these cities over the past three years by families from Southeast Asia and eastern Europe. The philosophy underlying Community Voices is that these populations can make significant contributions to the communities they become part of. Consistent with this notion, the facilitators emphasized a strengths-based approach to designing and managing the forums rather than a deficits-oriented one. The goal was to identify concrete strategies for translating strengths into specific interventions that could be developed and implemented by forum participants and others in the months following the event.

Your evaluation reveals, not surprisingly, that this ambitious effort has had mixed results. For example, some projects generated by the forums have thrived, whereas others have gone nowhere after an initial burst of enthusiasm. In the first draft of your evaluation report, you have tried to do justice to this reality, presenting both successes and failures in a balanced fashion. To add depth and richness to your presentation, you included a variety of quotations from the forum participants you interviewed. These quotes were selected to reflect the full range of positive–negative, success–failure experiences found in the evaluation.

You are now meeting with the foundation's senior program officer to review the draft, and he is not happy with your use of the quotes. In particular, he believes that most of the negative quotations are much too harsh and could influence readers to view the outcomes of Community Voices as less positive than is warranted, given *all* of the data presented in the report. Consequently, he would like you to either delete the offending quotes or replace them with other quotes that are less intensely negative.

You are not thrilled with the prospect of removing or replacing the quotes in question. You point out that a number of the *positive* quotations you cite in the report are, arguably, just as extreme (in the opposite direction) as the negative quotes that the program officer is taking issue with. Should those quotes be exchanged for less intense ones as well? Moreover, the number of relevant negative quotes you can choose from is relatively limited, making it difficult for you to satisfy the program officer's request even if you thought it was appropriate to do so.

The program officer does not find your response convincing. He claims that, in general, the harm done to a program by intense negative criticism outweighs the good that results from high praise. And the fact that there are fewer negative quotes than positive ones to choose from provides support, in his mind, for deemphasizing the significance of the negative comments.

Although you can appreciate the program officer's perspective, it's hard not to see this situation as, ultimately, just another instance in which a stakeholder wants an evaluation report to portray a program in a more positive light than is justified by the data. You are confident that you *have* written a fair, balanced report, and the quotations capture important truths—both positive and negative—about how certain subgroups of participants experienced the forums and their aftermath. The absolute number of negative quotes that you can choose from is, in the end, not the key issue here. You collected a great deal of other data in the evaluation (e.g., from surveys) that support your decision to use the quotes you've selected.

You know that Community Voices is a pet project of the senior program officer, and he has a lot invested in it emotionally and otherwise. But you are not going to let yourself be bullied in this situation. Is it possible for the two of you to reach a "meeting of the minds" on this issue?

QUESTIONS TO CONSIDER

1. Have you countered all of the senior program officer's arguments for not using the negative quotes you have chosen?

2. Would deleting *all* of the quotations from the report represent a compromise that you would consider in this case? What other compromises are possible? Are there any win–win solutions to this disagreement?

3. A time-honored piece of advice that has been offered in many contexts is, "Choose your battles carefully." Is a battle over the inclusion of certain quotations in your report one that is worth fighting? Why or why not?

4. In this scenario you are the associate director of evaluation. Would you seek support from your supervisor, the director of evaluation, in making your case to the senior program officer? What factors might influence your decision?

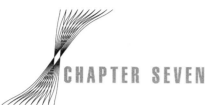

CHAPTER SEVEN

Utilization of Results

Nightly News

It's been nearly 5 hours since you turned off the 6:00 P.M. local news, and you're still agitated. The broadcast featured a story on a new community-based, substance abuse treatment program sponsored by the city's Health Department. The story included an excerpt from a press conference held by the mayor, in which she was effusive in her praise of this pilot program's effectiveness. The mayor indicated her desire to expand the program, so that "we can begin to turn the corner on drug abuse in our community."

You are a program evaluator in the Health Department and in that capacity had conducted an impact evaluation, including a cost–benefit analysis, of the program referred to by the mayor. In your view, the mayor played fast and loose with the facts when describing the results of your evaluation. For one thing, the program's impact on clients' subsequent substance abuse had been *extremely* modest. The mayor's remarks implied otherwise. Second, your cost–benefit analysis generated a ratio for the program of 1 to 0.58. That is, for every dollar spent on the program, the intervention returned 58 cents in benefits to society. Thus, from an economic perspective, the program did not represent a wise investment of resources. Implementing this intervention had turned out to be very expensive, and its efficacy was not strong enough to offset its considerable cost. The mayor had not mentioned the cost–benefit results in her televised comments. It was a love fest, pure and simple.

It's your opinion that a misrepresentation of evaluation results has occurred. Immediately after the broadcast you called your boss, who had attended the mayor's press conference and is the person in the Health Department to whom you had delivered your evaluation report. Perhaps the news clip had omitted comments from the mayor that presented a more realistic picture of the study's findings.

No such luck, according to your boss. "It's an election year, and the mayor wants to squeeze every possible ounce of positive PR out of this episode before November, which is only 2 months away. She knows that the program is too expensive to expand in the near future, so what will probably happen is that these announced plans will fade into the mist after the election, and the mayor will come up with a face-saving explanation somewhere down the line if she needs to." This response makes you very uncomfortable, and you proceed to share your concerns with your boss, concluding with the question, "What should we do?"

"Nothing," he replies. "What part of the word 'politics' don't you understand? We did *our* job. You conducted a competent evaluation and delivered it to me. I briefed the mayor *fully* on the results of the evaluation. She knows what you found. The mayor selected the aspects of the findings that she wanted to emphasize at the news conference. Strictly speaking, she didn't lie; this program *does* have a positive impact. Maybe she didn't tell the full story, but that's the norm in the political arena, not the exception. Do you really think the mayor would be willing to go before the public at this point and say, 'Oops, I didn't tell the whole truth'? I don't think so."

Four hours after the conversation with your boss, you don't feel better about any of this. No matter how you slice it, this boils down to a case of misrepresentation—substantively if not technically—and evaluators are not supposed to sit idly by when misrepresentation occurs. On the other hand, you're asking yourself, "Do I want to end up as a Don Quixote here, tilting at a windmill that could easily behead me?"

Fixing the Spin on Evaluation

Laura C. Leviton

Sooner or later most evaluators will encounter the sort of ethical dilemma posed in the Nightly News. To summarize, a Health Department program for drug treatment has been evaluated; the effects are positive but very small, and the program's high costs do not justify the expenditures. The mayor is facing reelection and cites the positive results as a reason to expand the program.

For those who practice evaluation for any length of time, it is inevitable that someone will use evaluation results selectively, misrepresent them (intentionally or unintentionally), or suppress relevant information. The Guiding Principle of Integrity/Honesty is very clear on this point: "Evaluators should not misrepresent their procedures, data or findings. Within reasonable limits, they should attempt to prevent or correct misuse of their work by others" (American Evaluation Association, 2004, Principle C-5). We should make sure that results are presented in accurate and complete form and interpreted correctly. But the devil is in the details: What on earth can be done in this particular case? What are the "reasonable limits"?

The scenario is particularly sensitive for at least two reasons. First, we presume that the mayor oversees the Health Department in which the evaluation was conducted and where the program resides. The evaluator, therefore, works for the mayor.[1] Second, the mayor has already gone public with a commitment to a position. For decades we have known that when individuals publicly take a stance, it is very unlikely that they will change their minds in response to additional information (Kiesler, 1971). It is especially difficult to modify the opinions of managers and public officials once they are publicly committed (Staw, 1976). And in an election year, it would be quite hard for the mayor to backtrack and be seen as waffling on the issues.

In this highly sensitive situation, the evaluator has a second responsibility, as outlined in the Guiding Principle of Responsibilities for General and Public Welfare: "Evaluators have obligations that encompass the public interest and good" (American Evaluation Association, 2004, Principle E-5). There are many considerations that are relevant to the public interest in addition to the use and misuse of an evaluation report. The *manner* in which evaluators correct misuse is extremely important, because it will have consequences for stake-holders, for the evaluator's credibility and effectiveness in other pro-jects, and for additional uses or misuses of the information. In other words, it is not only the evaluators' choices that have ethical dimen-sions but also the way in which they carry out those choices (Leviton, Needleman, & Shapiro, 1997). Of necessity, the Guiding Principles address the "what" of ethical choices but are silent on the "how." The evaluator needs to ask, "In this particular case, where does the greatest good lie? How can I address this problem in such a way as to best serve the public interest?"

THE EVALUATOR'S CHOICES

The evaluator has several options. To make the best decision in dealing with such a dilemma, evaluators should inquire about the details of the situation, making sure they understand the relevant facts, motiva-tions, and political positions.

Option 1: Keep Silent about the Misrepresented Results

This option is not in line with the principle of Responsibilities for Gen-eral and Public Welfare, which states that "freedom of information is essential in a democracy. Evaluators should allow all relevant stakeholders access to evaluative information. . . . Evaluators should actively disseminate information to stakeholders as resources allow" (American Evaluation Association, 2004, Principle E-3). Remaining silent would be comfortable in the short term but uncomfortable in the longer term. If the evaluator's boss is correct, the program could die a natural death after the election is over. In that case, no lasting harm to the city's resources will be incurred. However, there are no guarantees that the program will disappear. On the contrary, the program has all the markings of a pet project, and the mayor is committed publicly to supporting its expansion. Once the mayor is safely reelected, there may be few restraints on the program's expansion.

Remaining silent induces other harms. At a minimum, the evalua-tor's self-respect is damaged. In addition, the evaluator may need to draw a line in the sand: What future results will the evaluator's boss and the mayor decide to distort? Moreover, silence may simply not be necessary if the evaluator is protected by a civil service job. Thus, it may be that the mayor and supervisor cannot really do much if the evaluator pushes back in some way. But what is the best way to push back?

Option 2: Go Public with All the Information

The evaluator could hold a press conference and present the results in full, claiming that in the public interest a distorted picture needs to be corrected. But what good does that do? One of the Guiding Principles is satisfied and everything else falls apart! [2] Other harms are likely to flow from this action.

• The press would love the scandal, but they would focus on a cover-up, not on the merits of the case. It is unlikely that the press would convey the nuances of the results; more than likely they would simply report that the mayor distorted the conclusions and that the program does not really work. The evaluation results would become a political football, used rhetorically with no potential to improve the care of addicts in the city.

• Such an action indicates a great deal of disloyalty to the evaluator's organization. Loyalty as an ethical principle is not specifically covered in the Guiding Principles, but it is a principle nonetheless and should certainly guide our behavior.

• The Health Department could be seriously damaged by this action. Health departments have enough trouble as it is: They are embattled, underfunded, and underappreciated agencies that are essential to the public good (Leviton & Rhodes, 2005). Why damage maternal and child health services or immunization programs just because the mayor made a mistake?

• Perhaps the mayor is otherwise a good one. Is it worthwhile to publicly undermine her?

• Perhaps the Health Department relies on the evaluator for other important work. The evaluator's respect and credibility, or the chance for future credibility, disappear in a puff of smoke.

• Finally, there is the issue of the evaluator's employment. The Guiding Principles state that misrepresentation of results should be corrected *"where reasonable."* As community organizer Saul Alinsky once told a friend of mine, "Young man, you can't save the world if you can't feed your family."

Option 3: Leak the Results
to the Mayor's Political Opponent

See Option 2.

Option 4: Submit a Written Protest to the Supervisor
and Possibly the Mayor

This is the minimum required for acting with integrity in the situation. The Guiding Principles should be cited as a part of the letter. This might be sufficient to satisfy the need for "reasonable limits," in that the actions of these decision makers are largely beyond the evaluator's control. However, a written protest will not achieve a correct use of the results. It will, instead, polarize a situation that is better handled through Option 5.

Option 5: Push Back in Private
on the Health Department Supervisor
and, Preferably, the Mayor's Political Aides

This is the preferred option in most cases and the focus for the rest of this commentary. However, it must be done carefully, in such a way that the evaluator avoids the potential harms listed previously. The methods for the push-back become all important. Recommended reading for this purpose is *Getting to Yes* (Fisher & Ury, 1991), a classic text on negotiating from principle. Indeed, it is possible to use this situation to negotiate for more effective substance abuse treatment programs in the city.

A NEGOTIATED PUSH-BACK

Marshal Arguments

The evaluator should take several steps to see whether the mayor's unfortunate statement can be amended in some way. The first is to inquire whether the evaluation is a public document. The scenario does not make this clear. If the evaluation is publicly available, that is helpful because the mayor's political opponents will have access to the document as well. They will be looking for ways to criticize the mayor's positions. They can easily read the evaluation and, unless it is obscured by technical language, they are likely to see that the mayor presented only selected results to support a position. Indeed, the lack of cost savings to the public is potential political dynamite; the program is expensive, and it does not do very much! A clever opponent could readily portray the mayor's support of this program as coddling drug addicts at the expense of the taxpayer for little clear benefit.

FOIA Is Our Friend!

If the evaluation is not a public document, then the evaluator can point to the danger that it *could* be made public. The reason is that political foes and the press increasingly make use of the Freedom of Information Act (FOIA) in such cases. The evaluation and the report are publicly funded, making them potentially subject to disclosure.[3] The press will want news, or one television network will want to scoop the others.[4] Political opponents on a fishing expedition will be looking for areas to criticize the mayor. They might force the evaluation's public distribution before the election, because they are well aware that all evaluations have flaws. The program is very expensive and, therefore, a prime target. It is best for the mayor to be prepared. If she delays responding to a request for the report to be released, then the accusation will be that she has something to hide.

Make Allies

The evaluator also needs to know the political "lay of the land." The evaluator has a potential ally within the Health Department: the same supervisor who spoke so cynically about the use of the results. In general, health department professionals are very cognizant of the public interest and respectful of the need to present all the findings from a research study. For that reason, the supervisor cannot be overly pleased with the way the mayor has used the information. This same supervisor is ideal to serve as a bridge to the mayor and present the potential political problem that the report represents.

Does the mayor have handlers who are "spin doctors"? If so, will they recognize the dangers presented by the public availability of this evaluation? It is difficult to correct what spin doctors do when they legitimate a position through science, because many times they will not listen to caveats or problems. Often, it does not matter whether the spin doctor is the employer, a fellow employee elsewhere in the organization, or an outsider with an axe to grind—the spin doctor can be incorrigible.

The best course of action with spin doctors is to spell out clearly the political dangers of a public commitment to a position that will be untenable if the entire report is released. Certainly, the evaluator can also negotiate from principle, citing the Guiding Principles as grounds to release the entire report to the press and the taxpayers. However, it is the danger of public embarrassment that is likely to convince political operatives to backtrack, not the merits of the case. As Alinsky (1971) observed, "People will do the right thing for the wrong reasons."

Reframe the Issues

At this point, the mayor's aides will be looking for a way out. If the evaluator can get a foot in the mayor's door, he or she can assist both the Health Department supervisor and the mayor a great deal by reframing the results. In my experience, both interpretation and misinterpretation of evaluation findings are profoundly influenced by the user's frame of reference. The evaluator can provide a better frame of reference for the meaning of the results and help to avoid their misuse.

The city's community-based substance abuse intervention produced small positive effects. But what do those effects actually mean? First, the evaluator can convey exactly what the results signify for the number of substance abusers who stay clean and sober in the city—not all that many, apparently. By reviewing the literature on the effects of substance abuse treatment, the evaluator can translate these outcomes into likely impacts on city-wide employment and crime. Equally important, the evaluator can improve the mayor's frame of reference by comparing this program's costs and benefits with those reported in evaluations of similar programs elsewhere. From this vantage point, the outcomes of the city's pilot program will look increasingly paltry and unsatisfactory. Comparing the cost of the city's pilot program with the average cost of these other programs would also help ground the results in specifics that the mayor can use.

In fact, with proper preparation, the mayor's response is likely to be, "Why can't our program be as good as their programs? Sounds like we have some work to do!" The evaluator can point out that most startup programs gain efficiency as time goes on but that the program can definitely be strengthened, perhaps by incorporating the best practices that the evaluator has discovered through the literature review.

Fancy Footwork

The evaluator may want to suggest a preemptive release of the document and a bit of backtracking. Good politicians can retreat from untenable positions, even if they do not want to do so. One way the mayor could backtrack would be to use the reframed results as follows: "We are very pleased with the proof of the concept that this program has demonstrated. We have now shown that a community-based program of this kind is feasible and can produce positive impact. However, there is still work to do. When we compare the cost of the program with that of others in the nation, we are convinced that we can get even better results at lower cost. Therefore, we will be seeking guidance to improve the program as time goes on. I owe no less to the taxpayers of this city than to give them this splendid program, but to watch the cost as well."

WHAT SHOULD HAVE BEEN DONE BEFOREHAND

Involve Diverse Stakeholders to Prevent Misuse of Evaluation

It is noteworthy that the scenario does not include other stakeholders relevant to the program and its evaluation: treatment centers, community organizations, recovered substance abusers, concerned citizens, and community leaders. The Guiding Principles are explicit about the importance of consulting relevant stakeholders in the conduct and reporting of evaluations. It is the evaluator's responsibility, not the client's, to make sure that these stakeholders are involved. The Responsibilities for General and Public Welfare principle states that "when planning and reporting evaluations, evaluators should include relevant perspectives and interests of the full range of stakeholders" (American Evaluation Association, 2004, Principle E-1). In this scenario, much of the trouble could have been avoided by involving people and organizations outside of city government. These outside stakeholders would have access to the report, so they would be aware if the mayor used results selectively. If the mayor believed that the stakeholders had all read the report, she might not have misused the findings.

In reality, the early involvement of diverse stakeholders is highly compatible with the mayor's true political needs in this scenario. A variety of constituents would endorse the methods and the findings, making them less subject to criticism. Alternatively, the mayor and the Health Department would be aware of criticisms early in the life of the evaluation.

Early engagement of stakeholders also prepares them to better understand the results and use them appropriately. Although misuse and selective use are always possible, an informed and democratic debate about the findings is our best assurance that they will be used well. Political debates over such results do not usually cause the demise of a program. Instead, it is common for stakeholders to tinker with the program in an attempt to lower its cost and improve its effectiveness (Shadish, Cook, & Leviton, 1991).

Develop Trust and Credibility
to Prevent Misuse of Evaluations

I know of several cases in which an internal evaluator helped a political official avoid publicly supporting policies or programs that were deemed ineffective on the basis of research. In these instances, the evaluator first built credibility with the official in every way possible. One evaluator for a school system established credibility during the energy crisis of the late 1970s by staying in school basements to monitor energy usage. That same evaluator was then able to go privately to the school's superintendent and board to advise them against a policy they were about to announce. He had evidence that it would be ineffective and even harmful to students, and he convinced them of this. Another researcher has a long-standing relationship with the state's governor and has supported him in political campaigns. He was able to advise the governor to abandon a highly flawed policy, but did so behind the scenes.

In the Nightly News scenario, the evaluator was not in a position to build trust directly with the mayor. However, the evaluator could develop stronger credibility with the Health Department supervisor. Ideally, the evaluator would have accompanied the supervisor to brief the mayor on the results of the evaluation. Indeed, in a relationship of trust, the evaluator might have cautioned the supervisor that the results were somewhat complex; seeing that the mayor was facing reelection soon, she would want to avoid some pitfalls of interpretation. As the Guiding Principle of Responsibilities for General and Public Welfare asserts, "In all cases, evaluators should strive to present results clearly and simply so that clients and other stakeholders can easily understand the evaluation process and results" (American Evaluation Association, 2004, Principle E-3).

CONCLUSION

The evaluator in this scenario is not powerless by any means. At a minimum, actions can be taken to satisfy the Guiding Principles. But more than the minimum is feasible and desirable: The mayor can be guided to a more tenable position. However, a positive outcome depends on the evaluator's political skill and political capital. To prevent future problems, the evaluator needs to build trust and credibility and to involve the key stakeholders in the evaluation.

NOTES

1. Many health departments actually work for an appointed board of health and are quasi-independent from other branches of city government.
2. An acquaintance of mine once held a press conference to correct misstatements on a nonevaluation issue. The headline the next day read: "Everyone Is Lying but Me." The press conference did not achieve his purpose.
3. The FOIA applies to federally funded programs. However, many states have their own FOI legislation.
4. The media in Little Rock, Arkansas frequently use FOIA to scoop each other about statewide news. A colleague there has to be extremely careful about the completion of evaluation reports and the timing of their release in order to prevent a premature release and potential misuse of the information.

REFERENCES

Alinsky, S. (1971). *Rules for radicals.* New York: Random House.

American Evaluation Association. (2004). *Guiding principles for evaluators* (rev.). Available at *www.eval.org/Publications/GuidingPrinciples.asp.*

Fisher, R., & Ury, W. L. (1991). *Getting to yes: Negotiating agreement without giving in.* New York: Penguin.

Kiesler, C. A. (1971). *The psychology of commitment: Experiments linking behavior to belief.* New York: Academic Press.

Leviton, L. C., Needleman, C. E., & Shapiro, M. (1997). *Confronting public health risks: A decision maker's guide.* Thousand Oaks, CA: Sage.

Leviton, L. C., & Rhodes, S. D. (2005). Public health: Policy, practice, and perceptions. In A. R. Kovner, J. R. Knickman, & S. Jonas (Eds.), *Health care delivery in the United States* (8th ed., pp. 90–129). New York: Springer.

Shadish, W. R., Cook, T. D., & Leviton, L. C. (1991). *Foundations of program evaluation: Theories of practice.* Newbury Park, CA: Sage.

Staw, B. (1976). Knee-deep in the big muddy: A study of escalating commitment to a chosen course of action. *Organizational Behavior and Human Performance, 16,* 27–44.

COMMENTARY

From Substance Use to Evaluation Misuse: Is There a Way Out?

Sharon F. Rallis

As the lead evaluator who conducted the study of the substance abuse treatment program sponsored by the city's Health Department, I have encountered an ethical "situation." The mayor has publicly misrepresented the evaluation's findings, making the program seem more effective than it actually is. My boss tells me that there is nothing I can do because the evaluation has fallen into the political arena where power rules over truth. I am deeply unsettled and wonder how I should respond, or should I respond at all? I look back at my graduate courses on ethics and realize that such problems don't have cut-and-dry solutions. I cannot seek *the* answer. Instead, I must reason my way through this, drawing on my intuition, personal values, the standards within my profession, and moral principles. This commentary follows my path through each of these domains.

INTUITION

My intuition tells me that the mayor's misrepresentation of findings is not right, but my intuition also signals that I would be a fool to intervene. What would I accomplish? Who would hear me? I realize that my chances of being heard were much better earlier in the process, as the evaluation's approach and conditions were being negotiated, especially in terms of the project's scope and use of results. The next time I will know to be more thorough in my negotiations, sensitive to various stakeholders' interests and anticipating political consequences. But that time has passed. One powerful stakeholder, the mayor, has already taken action and reported her interpretation of the findings. She has the power of the symbolic on her side; that is, the program she describes is fighting a social evil and thus is seen as desirable. The public believes in what they perceive to be her program and believes in her as a crusader against the scourge of drug use. Any public action I take now would be too late, given that she has framed the issue in her terms and not on all the data. Should I raise my voice to counter her words, I will indeed be playing the role of Don Quixote, Ineffective Intervener.

PERSONAL VALUES

On the other hand, my values run counter to inaction. I am an evaluator because I want my work to be used, specifically in the service of social improvement (see Smith, 1978). I want to make a positive difference. The city's Health Department initiated the substance abuse program in response to an identified need in the community, and tax dollars have been allocated to program implementation. I saw evaluating the program's effects as a way to get information to decision makers so they can most effectively address the problem of drug abuse in the city. I wrote my report and delivered my findings, but I do not feel I have completed my job as evaluator (despite what my boss says) until I see the information used. Evaluation entails more than simply producing and delivering a report, so I had hoped to present the findings to personnel related to the program both in the field and in the mayor's office.

Unfortunately, my intended communications about the quality of the program have been short-circuited. I had scheduled a meeting with the director of the treatment program for later in the week to review the findings so we could consider what aspects of the program were worth retaining as well as what other options existed. The dubious quality of the program, in terms of its merit (modest results) and worth (not a wise investment; costs exceed the return), would have been apparent. We could have considered action strategies. But, thus far, I have only had the opportunity to provide a textual representation of the findings, in the form of my recently submitted report, which quickly found its way to the mayor. Had I a chance for dialogue with the program director and mayor prior to the press conference, I might have been able to break through the politics (see Rallis & Rossman, 2001).

Now the mayor has *used* my work but certainly not in the way I had intended (Patton, 1997). I must ask myself, What is the impact of this use? I see the impact as purely political. As my boss noted, once the pressure of the election year diminishes, the mayor will probably let plans for program expansion die. I want the program replaced with one that better serves those in need of treatment, so this outcome conflicts with my personal values. Regrettably, the evaluation will not be used effectively to address the drug problem in the community; it is instead being employed to make the mayor look good. How can I look *myself* in the mirror knowing that my work has provided fodder for a conniving politician?

PROFESSIONAL STANDARDS

Where did I go wrong? I turn to my professional resource for ethical practice, the Guiding Principles for Evaluators (American Evaluation Association, 2004). The relevance of several aspects of the Guiding Principles is obvious. The first principle, Systematic Inquiry, raises the issue of whether I conducted a systematic, data-based study. Yes, I did adhere to the highest technical standards, and I worked closely with the program administrator to frame questions and choose a workable approach. I see myself as a critical friend (Rallis & Rossman, 2000) of the program leadership, so that together we can interpret and critique the process and results. But therein lies a problem: I worked with stakeholders only at the *program* level. Including the mayor in these deliberations seemed premature and excessive. Even in retrospect, the notion of trying to involve her early in the process strikes me as cumbersome and impractical. I doubt I would have had access to her during the early stages, and by the time the mayor was interested, it was too late to ensure her understanding and shared interpretation.

The Competence principle, which requires that my evaluation team and I possess the skills and experience, including cultural competence, to employ appropriate strategies for the evaluation, is not at issue here. Indeed, my team's reputation for competence and culturally sensitive evaluations may have been a factor in the mayor's choice to use our evaluation results. The team is composed of a diverse mix of seasoned evaluators, and two of us have more than a decade of experience evaluating substance abuse programs. Furthermore, we have an advisory council that includes recovered substance abusers. Who would dispute a report coming out of such a department?

The next principle, Integrity/Honesty, raises questions about our evaluation process. Although I believe we did display honesty and integrity in our own behavior, what did we do to ensure the honesty and integrity of the entire evaluation process? Because use of results *is* part of the process, I recognize that we fell short on this principle. Were the program leaders and clients aware of the potentially politically charged nature of the program? Could we have done anything different in our design, our negotiations, and our reporting to forestall the misrepresentation of the results? With hindsight, I can say that we may not have been transparent enough. I see that we should have scheduled opportunities to explain how the evaluation was being conducted and to share the results directly with various stakeholders, including the public. Had we publicized the evaluation from the start, the mayor might not have been able to hijack the dissemination of findings.

As an evaluator who believes she acts ethically, I hold the fourth principle, Respect for People, as paramount. This principle posits that evaluators must respect the security, dignity, and self-worth of respondents, program participants, clients, and other evaluation stakeholders. Concerning the respondents, I was vigilant regarding confidentiality and informed consent. But it is also my responsibility to "maximize the benefits and reduce any unnecessary harms that might occur" from the evaluation (American Evaluation Association, 2004, Principle D-3). Thus, I must ask myself, Who might be harmed by the mayor's actions?

Program participants (i.e., substance abusers) are hurt because they will be denied an improved or better program. The Health Department is unlikely to seek out another program because the mayor has represented this one as effective. Worse still, even this program will, as my boss predicts, fade into the mist of the political landscape because of its high costs. So program participants *are* harmed, and program participants are often from traditionally underrepresented and disempowered groups. I am faced with another example of those in power and of the dominant culture defining what is best for others and limiting their access to services. I am shirking my responsibility to those in need of an intervention if I do not rebut the mayor's praise of the current treatment program.

What other clients or stakeholders must be respected? Program leadership is harmed in this instance because my goal of providing information to guide program improvement or choice of program alternatives is jeopardized. The mayor's declaration of the current program's effectiveness dilutes the power of Health Department officials to modify this program or propose another intervention. That their work has been harmed offers an additional reason for me to take action to counter the mayor's misrepresentation.

Another group of stakeholders moves us into the final Guiding Principle, Responsibilities for General and Public Welfare. As the mayor made clear, the community does have a drug problem. Without effective programs to address this issue that affects, directly or indirectly, the welfare of all citizens, the community as a whole suffers. And because the program is not cost effective, dollars sunk into it are not a wise investment. Thus, citizens as taxpayers are harmed if expenditures of tax dollars continue toward this costly and ineffective intervention.

However, is not the mayor also a stakeholder? Does she have rights that I must respect? This question leads me to another level of reasoning: the moral credibility of one's actions. My values tell me that the mayor's actions are not defensible. Still, as my boss made clear, her selective use of the findings is the norm in the political arena. The public sees her as a good leader, and she has made progress in other areas that are seen important, such as rebuilding sections of the city to attract businesses and bring in more jobs. So, my boss asks, What purpose does it serve to challenge her? Might doing so weaken her in other areas where she has been effective? Thus, might not my challenge be wrong?

MORAL PRINCIPLES

I am left to examine the moral defensibility of my own behavior: Should I follow my boss's directive and let it go? Or do I have an obligation to act and ensure that the full story of the program's shortcomings be told and heard? I said that I aim to be an ethical evaluator, and I hold "ethics" to be *standards for conduct based on moral principles.* What moral principles, then, can guide my reasoning?

First, there are the *ethics of consequences,* also known as *utilitarianism:* "the doctrine that the greatest good of the greatest number should be the guiding principle of conduct" (*Oxford English Dictionary,* 1993, p. 3534). This doctrine, elaborated in the late 18th and early 19th centuries by philosophers such as Hume and Mill, approves actions that benefit the majority. As an evaluator, I do not find this ethic helpful because it could support arguments for both speaking out and remaining silent, depending on one's perspective. If you see the majority as benefiting from an effective substance abuse program, utilitarianism would urge me to share my concerns. In contrast, were you to see the majority as benefiting from the mayor retaining her office, utilitarianism would seek to stifle my voice.

Kant's *ethic of individual rights and responsibilities* provides an additional perspective (1788/1956). Kant emphasizes the unconditional value of human beings, positing that each person deserves to be treated as an end, not as a means to an end. When I think of the individual drug abusers in the community who need help, I see them as an end in themselves, *not* as a means to the mayor's reelection. Thus, I must speak out.

At the same time, I must consider my department and the evaluation team. Do I not have a responsibility to them and their rights? If I voice my concerns, they might be hurt through association with me. Still, any harm team members experience would be a side effect because I am not using them as a means to an end. I suspect Kant would recommend that I act as I would want others to act. But that *is* my problem: I know what I wish the mayor had done, but I cannot figure out how I would want an evaluator to act. What is the ethical action? Which moral principle applies?

It seems that I may have returned to *utilitarianism*. However, I remain unsatisfied because this doctrine seems unfair in this instance. What if only a few drug users are harmed because this ineffective program continues until it dies its own political death, while the majority of the public benefits from the reelection of the mayor? Do not those few matter? The *ethic of justice* applied here moves my reasoning forward. According to Rawls (1971), the benefit or welfare of the least advantaged, not that of the majority or the average, must drive my decision. In his view, improving the welfare of the least advantaged, no matter how few in number, ultimately benefits everyone in the long term. As Chief Roberta Jamieson (2005) of Canada's National Aboriginal Achievement Foundation has exhorted evaluators, we need to ask ourselves what impact our actions might have on the "seventh generation." Following this reasoning, my decision is clear: I should respond to the needs of the substance abusers, because ignoring them puts the community and its future generations in jeopardy. I must speak out so that the truth of the program is known and a more effective program can be put in place.

Is speaking out a simplistic solution? Will voicing my concerns mean that an improved or effective program will be instituted? According to my boss, the answer is no. But I have reasoned that I must do *something*. The moral principles I have been discussing tend toward universal laws and generalizations: what we want everyone to do; what benefits the most; what abstract individual rights call for. I need a principle that will guide me in this instance, at this time, with this program, with these participants, and with this mayor. The *ethic of caring* offers a workable answer as it directs me to focus on the context of this specific case. Noddings (1984) and Gilligan (1982) encourage me to look at the relationships between those experiencing *this particular situation*. Whatever action I take must consider the needs and interests of these participants as they relate to each other and must enable resources to be directed toward continuing the relationships between the various interests. I must recognize that the interests of the program staff, program participants, the mayor, and the community are intertwined. What does that mean in terms of action by me, the evaluator whose report was misused?

Through the *caring* lens, I see that the mayor's words, once spoken, do not necessarily signify the end of my evaluation's use and impact. They do not necessarily prevent improvements to the current substance abuse program or adoption of a new and better program. I may actually be able to use the dramatic attention brought to the evaluation for the program's benefit. After all, the mayor did confirm the existence of the drug problem in the city and that the program does have positive aspects. I will keep my appointment with the program director. We will discuss what the Health Department needs in order to run a successful and cost-effective substance abuse program, based on what the evaluation discovered. We will identify ways, again based on the evaluation findings, to get what is needed.

In addition, I will assume that the mayor does want to "turn the corner on drug abuse in our community" (as she announced in the press conference), so I will try to schedule an appointment with her, referring to this statement and indicating that my purpose in talking with her is to generate ways to support her espoused desires to build on this success. Although the mayor is unlikely to meet with me herself, she will almost certainly have relevant aides do so, because this would be politically to her advantage. I will suggest that the program director and possibly Health Department leadership join us. We will discuss how the city can continue to support substance abuse treatment with more cost-effective returns, using information embedded in the report and ideas produced during my conversation with the program director about the evaluation findings.

What I am doing with my more collaborative and participatory approach is neither to cave in to power nor to tilt at windmills. Rather, I have regrounded myself in what I believe are the purposes and uses of evaluation. After all, Cronbach et al. (1980) state that evaluation is "better used to understand events and processes for the sake of guiding future activities" than employed to look back "in order to assign praise or blame" (p. 4). In their view, the evaluator is an educator whose success is judged by what others learn. As the evaluator in the

Nightly News case, I can enlighten discussion of alternative plans for social action. I am not so naïve as to expect that improvements will occur immediately, but I do believe that a more effective substance abuse program will result. After all, that is my idea of what an ethical evaluator's job is—to influence positive change through providing information for decision making—and I can best do so by building relationships among the various interests within the system.

REFERENCES

American Evaluation Association. (2004). *Guiding principles for evaluators* (rev.). Available at *www.eval.org/Publications/GuidingPrinciples.asp*.

Cronbach, L. J., Ambron, S. R., Dornbusch, S. M., Hess, R. D., Hornik, R. C., Phillips, D. C., et al. (1980). *Toward reform of program evaluation*. San Francisco: Jossey-Bass.

Gilligan, C. (1982). *In a different voice: Psychological theory and women's development*. Cambridge, MA: Harvard University Press.

Jamieson, R. (2005, October). *Diplomacy, democracy, and indigenous peoples*. Plenary address presented at the annual meeting of the American Evaluation Association, Toronto, Ontario, Canada.

Kant, I. (1956). *Critique of practical reason* (L. W. Beck, Trans.). New York: Liberal Arts Press. (Original work published 1788)

Noddings, N. (1984). *Caring: A feminine approach to ethics and moral education*. Berkeley: University of California Press.

Oxford English Dictionary (Vol. 1). (1993). Oxford, UK: Clarendon.

Patton, M. Q. (1997). *Utilization focused evaluation: The new century text* (3rd ed.). Thousand Oaks, CA: Sage.

Rallis, S. F., & Rossman, G. B. (2000). Dialogue for learning: Evaluator as critical friend. In R. Hopson (Ed.), *How and why language matters in evaluation* (New directions for evaluation, no. 86, pp. 81–92). San Francisco: Jossey-Bass.

Rallis, S. F., & Rossman, G. B. (2001). Communicating quality and qualities: The role of the evaluator as critical friend. In A. P. Benson, D. M. Hinn, & C. Lloyd (Eds.), *Visions of quality: How evaluators define, understand, and represent program quality* (pp. 107–120). Oxford, UK: JAI Press.

Rawls, J. (1971). *A theory of justice*. Cambridge, MA: Harvard University Press.

Smith, N. L. (1978). *The kinds of knowledge required for discipline-level assessment of evaluation methodology*. Portland, OR: Northwest Regional Educational Laboratory.

■   ■   ■   ■

WHAT IF . . . ?

. . . your boss specifically instructs you not to pursue the matter any further unless invited to do so by him or a representative of the mayor's office?

. . . your boss, in an interview published in a local newspaper a few days later, characterizes the results of the program evaluation in the same way that the mayor did?

. . . the program's impact had actually been quite positive, but that the mayor had significantly understated its effectiveness in her press conference, indicating that the Health Department would continue to search for viable interventions in the substance abuse treatment domain?

FINAL THOUGHTS

Nightly News

In the opinion of the two commentators addressing the Nightly News scenario, responding with silence to the mayor's misrepresentation of evaluation results is not an option. The crucial challenge Leviton and Rallis face is finding an effective way to voice their concerns. Moral indignation does not provide a blueprint for successful intervention, and evaluators must be careful not to let the strong emotions that accompany indignation result in impulsive actions that can generate short-term satisfaction but long-term failure. Thus, it is not surprising that both commentators advocate a collaborative strategy of reaching out to constituencies within the Health Department and the mayor's office. In essence, the message being communicated is an offer of help: "How can we use *all of our knowledge* about this program to serve the interests of program participants and staff, taxpayers, the mayor, and indeed the community as a whole?" Such an approach is likely to generate more positive outcomes than a confrontational, exposé-oriented strategy.

Leviton and Rallis also agree that the misrepresentation in this case might have been prevented with more thorough involvement of a variety of stakeholders throughout the evaluation. At the very least, the mayor probably would have thought twice (or maybe even three times) before portraying the study's findings as she did, knowing that a bevy of well-informed stakeholders was looking over her shoulder.

The analysis of Rallis is distinctive in that she explicitly refers to several well-known schools of philosophical thought: Mill's utilitarianism, Kant's ethic of individual rights and responsibilities, Rawls's ethic of justice, and Noddings's ethic of caring. She indicates that, in the end, it is the ethic of caring that is most useful to her in determining what the evaluator should do in the Nightly News scenario. Readers should consider for themselves the implications for the case of these different philosophical perspectives to see whether they come to the same conclusions as Rallis.

Finally, the commentaries of Leviton and Rallis leave at least one tantalizing question unanswered: How should you respond if your collaborative overture is rebuffed? What if no one in the Health Department or the mayor's office is receptive to your collegial attempt to view, and use, the evaluation's findings in a more productive fashion? Have you met your ethical obligations in the situation by making the effort, or is a more contentious, whistle-blowing approach now called for? What would you do? And why?

Is My Job Done Yet?

It's been nearly 4 months since you completed a debriefing meeting with the director and assistant director of human resources (HR) at a high-profile regional bank where you had conducted a process evaluation of the bank's Employee Assistance Program (EAP). The bank contracts with an external provider for EAP services, and you are an external evaluator not affiliated with the provider. Although your primary client is the HR director, you were recruited for the project by the assistant director, whom you have known since college.

Among the EAP-related concerns voiced by employees during the evaluation were the following:

- Suspicions that the confidentiality of employees using the EAP had occasionally been violated by the service provider.
- Complaints that the service periods covered under the EAP were too short to be of significant help for certain types of problems.
- Perceptions of bureaucratic obstacles that made it difficult for employees to access the program quickly and easily.
- A more generalized belief that the managerial culture of the bank discouraged employees, both subtly and not so subtly, from taking advantage of the EAP.

In both your written report and the debriefing, you noted that, in your judgment, these concerns were serious and that failing to address them could eventually damage the EAP's credibility beyond repair. You expressed your willingness to facilitate a limited number of follow-up meetings with bank employees, managers, and representatives of the service provider to discuss the evaluation's results. The director thanked you for your offer and indicated that he would definitely keep it in mind as he dealt with the implications of the report in the weeks and months to come.

You have not heard from the director since then, but this afternoon you had a chance encounter with the assistant director, who informed you that, as far as she could tell, the director had done nothing with the evaluation. Indeed, a number of employees had asked the assistant director about the fate of the evaluation. Several employees even claimed that, increasingly, the "word on the street" was that the evaluator was a friend and ally of the director who had been brought in to placate employees in the short run and that the director had never intended to be truly responsive to their concerns about the EAP.

The assistant director wonders if there is anything that *you* can do to salvage the impact of the evaluation. And she is upset that you are apparently being viewed negatively by some of the employees who participated in the study.

You, too, are distressed at how things have unfolded, but you are not sure what you're in a position to do at this point. You've already made an explicit offer to the director to assist with follow-up, but he has not pursued it. Is it really appropriate for you to do anything else? And if so, what might that be?

QUESTIONS TO CONSIDER

1. Would the Guiding Principles support you in taking action in this case? Would they *require* you to take action in this case?

2. Does the alleged "whispering campaign" among employees that is damaging to your professional reputation provide justification for you to intervene after the evaluation has been completed?

3. Are there any steps you could have taken earlier in the evaluation to minimize the likelihood of these problematic events occurring?

4. If the evaluation had discovered *confirmed* instances of confidentiality violation by the service provider, would that affect your decision about whether, and how, to respond to the director's apparent inaction?

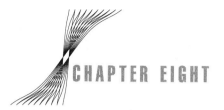

CHAPTER EIGHT

Lessons Learned

Extracting ethical lessons from case scenarios is a challenging task. One runs the risk of learning too much or too little. The "too much" can occur if one overgeneralizes. Every scenario is unique. Changing one or two details in a case can significantly alter the ethical terrain that the evaluator must negotiate. As Strike et al. (2002) observe, "No matter how much information is presented [in a case], it will be possible to imagine another fact that might change our minds" (p. xiii). Thus, applying, in a template-like fashion, the lessons of one scenario to another is likely to result in important differences between the two situations being overlooked. Newcomers to evaluation are especially vulnerable to such missteps.

The "too little" can result if one overreacts to instances in which commentators disagree on how the evaluator should deal with the problems presented by the case. The temptation here is to throw up one's hands and complain that scenarios represent little more than ink blots for commentators' personal values and prejudices. To be sure, in two instances, the recommendations offered by our commentators differed sharply (The Coordination Project and The Folder). In two others, there was at least partial disagreement (The Damp Parade and Mainstream). This leaves two scenarios characterized by consensus (Knock, Knock, What's There? and Nightly News). However, this state of affairs simply reflects the variation that can be found among evaluators in the real world when they encounter ethical challenges in their work (see also Datta, 2002; Morris & Jacobs, 2000). Strike et al. (2002) note that "in ethics, little is ever quite so obvious that reasonable people cannot disagree" (p. ix). One can view such an outcome as an indication of the *strength* of case scenarios, not a weakness. Specifically, they can help us explore the diverse influences, including but not limited to professional guidelines, that contribute to an evaluator's response to a given ethical conflict. Indeed, it might be argued that this represents the primary value of case analysis, at least in the domain of ethics. With this background in mind, let us examine some of the themes and implications that emerge from the cases and commentaries in this volume.

THE VALUE OF THE GUIDING PRINCIPLES

Given Chapter One's discussion of the strengths and limitations of professional guidelines, we should not be surprised to find that the Guiding Principles are useful for dissecting ethical challenges in evaluation. It is noteworthy that, when the pairs of commentaries are considered together, each case was examined from the perspective of all five Guiding Principles. Overall, these analyses constitute detailed, persuasive testimony that the principles have substantial value for analyzing the ethical issues raised by a given scenario.

On the other hand, the Guiding Principles do not necessarily provide an "answer sheet" for how to respond to specific problems. Indeed, it is hard to escape Datta's conclusion, based on her analysis of commentaries in the Ethical Challenges section of the *American Journal of Evaluation*, that "the [Guiding] Principles in particular seem so open to interpretation that a wide range of values, preferences, and opinions can be projected onto them" (2002, p. 195). As we have seen, application of the principles did not guarantee that pairs of commentators would reach identical, or even overlapping, conclusions about what the evaluator should do. This is the price that is paid when guidelines are "intentionally couched in very general terms" (Shadish, this volume, p. 134).

The generality of the Guiding Principles should not obscure their utility for conducting an in-depth analysis of a specific evaluation's ethical dimensions. Commentators made impressive use of various subsections of the principles in crafting their responses to the cases. Of course, one can speculate about the sequence of events operating here. Did the detailed application of the principles precede or follow the commentator's judgment concerning what actions the evaluator should take? The former sequence, dubbed "structural use" by Datta (2002), is more consistent with our idealized vision of how the Guiding Principles should be employed. Given the myriad factors that influence the process of human reasoning, a definitive answer to this question is probably not possible. The more crucial question is, To what extent do the Guiding Principles provide a meaningful framework and catalyst for reflecting on ethical issues in evaluation, even if they do not lead to a single decision-making end point? In that respect, the richness of the commentaries suggests that the value of the Guiding Principles is significant.

THE IMPORTANCE OF THE ENTRY/CONTRACTING PHASE

Generally speaking, *preventing* ethical problems is preferable to having to respond to them once they occur. In the scenarios on which ethical difficulties manifested themselves after the entry/contracting phase had concluded, commentators frequently discussed actions the evaluator could have taken during that initial stage to forestall subsequent conflicts. Our knowledge of ethical challenges in evaluation has developed to the point at which we can generate well-educated guesses about the types of problems a particular evaluation is likely to be vulnerable to (see Chapter One). And as Morris (2003) observes, "The more thoroughly these matters are discussed at the beginning of the evaluation, the less likely they will arise in problematic fashion later on. And if they *do* arise, a framework for addressing them has at least been established" (p. 319).

The message here is ultimately a simple one: Conversations that take place early, even if they are somewhat tense and uncomfortable, can minimize the need for much more tense and uncomfortable conversations (and actions) later. Evaluators can use these interactions to acquaint key stakeholders with the most relevant aspects of the Guiding Principles and the Program Evaluation Standards. For example, if an evaluator suspects that a politically volatile study might lead to strong pressures to distort findings in a final report, these concerns could be shared with the appropriate parties within a context that emphasizes the evaluator's ethical and professional responsibilities. Would this action eliminate all attempts at undue influence? Probably not. But, having employed such a strategy, the evaluator is likely to be in a stronger position to counter these attempts should they occur.

Of course, it is not possible to anticipate every type of ethical problem that might emerge in an evaluation, no matter how thorough we are in our initial discussions with stakeholders. However, this is no excuse for failing to develop, in collaboration with stakeholders, an explicit understanding of how, at least at a general level, ethical concerns should be handled. The entry/contracting stage of the evaluation is the ideal time to do this, and excellent resources are available, many from the consulting literature, to help evaluators manage the process (e.g., Block, 2000). Facilitating such a discussion is an excellent way of setting the stage for a *metaevaluation* of the project, in which one monitors and reviews the extent to which the evaluation embodies the principles of sound evaluation practice, ethically and otherwise (see the Metaevaluation Standard of the second edition of the Program Evaluation Standards; Joint Committee on Standards for Educational Evaluation, 1994, pp. 185–190). Metaevaluation represents a powerful mechanism for enhancing the overall quality of evaluation.

THE ENGAGEMENT OF STAKEHOLDERS

Identifying and working with relevant stakeholders is a bedrock task in virtually any evaluation. It is also a crucial step in confronting ethical conflicts, at least in the opinion of most of our commentators. At first glance, this point may appear so intuitively obvious that one might question whether it is worth making. However, the anxiety-provoking nature of ethical challenges can frequently prompt individuals, including evaluators, to try to resolve them "in private." That is, the evaluator sees the problem as an "undiscussable" (Argyris, 1985) that should not be shared with others until he or she has reached a decision about how the problem should be solved. Evaluators who adopt such an approach are *not* prone to engage stakeholders as they work through ethical quandaries. This results in the loss of information and perspectives that could be extremely valuable in resolving the conflict. Indeed, in some instances, it may even contribute to the evaluator believing that an ethical problem exists when, in fact, there is none.

Evaluators need to be skilled at using open-ended questions rather than position statements to raise ethical issues with stakeholders. This approach tends to minimize stakeholder defensiveness and maximize the potential solutions that can be brought to bear on the problem. Faced with pressure to delete a controversial finding from a report, a response of "I can't do that because . . . " is less likely to generate a productive interaction than one that begins with "What is it about this finding that makes you feel it shouldn't be included?" or "What would be the positive *and* negative consequences of omitting this result?" To be sure, the evaluator may need to take a firm stand at some point if the situation is so clear-cut that the implications of professional standards or personal values are unambiguous. But if Chavis (this volume, p. 53) is correct in asserting that a relationship "based on respect and mutual learning" is vital for evaluations to succeed, then both evaluators and stakeholders are better served, in the long run, when their interactions begin with more questions and fewer declarations.

THE EVALUATOR'S CONTRIBUTION TO THE CONFLICT

As has been noted, most of us are not inclined to see our own behavior as causing the problems we encounter, and there is no compelling reason to believe that evaluators are immune to this tendency. Indeed, the commentators often explored how the evaluator's actions (or inaction) played, at the very least, a "supporting role" in the ethical predicament in which the evaluator found him- or herself. It is important to note that this is not synonymous with claiming that the evaluator behaved unethically (although it is certainly possible for evaluators to do so). Rather, the point being made is that the evaluator's conduct increased the likelihood that ethical challenges would emerge. For example, failing to develop a shared understanding of confidentiality during the entry/contracting or design phase can produce serious problems later in the evaluation.

When these situations arise, a lack of defensiveness on the evaluator's part becomes crucial. Although this can be difficult to achieve, it is the same request that evaluators typically make of stakeholders when ethical conflicts occur. To the degree that evaluators model nondefensive behavior, the chances that stakeholders will respond "in kind" are bolstered. And this can only bode well for problem resolution.

PERSONAL VALUES AND CULTURAL COMPETENCE

We do not wait until we become evaluators to develop values that influence our behavior. By the time we encounter the Guiding Principles or the Program Evaluation Standards, we have accumulated a whole host of ideas about what ethical conduct requires. Clearly articulating these ideas and understanding how they relate to professional guidelines and the professional challenges one faces are essential tasks for any evaluator. Our commentators sometimes went to great lengths to explain how "who they are," in terms of their personal identity and values, interacted with the scenarios they were analyzing (e.g., Kirkhart, davis).

A major reason for the importance of this self-examination relates to cultural competence, as Kirkhart indicates. Surfacing one's taken-for-granted values and unstated assumptions, which so often have cultural roots, is necessary if evaluators are going to place into proper perspective their views of stakeholders and settings. This is more than just an issue of being competent in a narrow, technical sense; the distinctive cultural contexts that evaluators encounter can conflict with their *ethical* sensibilities (see Paasche-Orlow, 2004). How far should evaluators extend themselves in adapting to these environments in order to "successfully" carry out a study? There are no easy answers.

At the most general level, decisions to accept or decline an evaluation project can be affected by this self-reflection. ("Am I ethically comfortable in evaluating a program sponsored by an organization with this particular value-based agenda?") Once an evaluation is undertaken, personal values can influence one's response to numerous features of the project—for example, ways in which specific stakeholder groups (e.g., females, youth, the elderly, racial/ethnic minorities, religious fundamentalists, the disabled) are treated or the degree to which one feels justified in drawing generalized conclusions from evaluation data. Distinguishing between what professional guidelines in evaluation require of you and what *you* require of you can be a challenging endeavor because the latter often shapes our interpretation of the former. Indeed, this can be the source of disagreements among evaluators about what the ethical practice of evaluation requires. Long-standing controversies focused on evaluators' responsibilities in the domains of stakeholder participation and evaluation utilization (Morris, 2003) are just two of the arenas where it might be argued that personal ethics, philosophical/ideological preferences, and professional standards have interacted in ways that complicate (or "enrich," depending on one's perspective) ethical analysis in evaluation. As the field matures, evaluation theorists and practitioners will continue to explore and, it is hoped, clarify these relationships.

THINKING ..., THINKING ABOUT DOING ..., AND DOING

Systematically examining ethical challenges that evaluators encounter ("thinking") is a major goal of this volume, and our commentators certainly provide a wealth of analysis in that regard. They also offer recommendations for action, sometimes laying out step-by-step strategies in considerable detail (e.g., Kirkhart, Cooksy, Barrington). This can be described as the "thinking about doing" dimension. Of course, if the scenarios were real situations rather than hypothetical vignettes, the evaluators in them would be faced with the task of putting into practice these recommendations, the "doing" dimension. The "doing" can be daunting for at least two reasons. In some cases, the actions may require knowledge or skills that the evaluator does not possess (or does not *believe* that he or she possesses; e.g., knowledge of state-of-the-art data-analysis techniques or skills in facilitating constructive interactions between conflicting stakeholder groups). In the short run, these obstacles can be intimidating, but in the long term they are best seen as technical matters to be addressed as one expands one's evaluation-related competencies.

The other source of difficulty is the personal and/or professional risks that doing the ethically right thing might entail. Hendricks speaks pointedly to this issue in his commentary on The Folder scenario, noting that:

> The Guiding Principles allow me no latitude to withhold important information simply because sharing it might make my job more difficult. In fact, several Guiding Principles clearly urge me to share all relevant information without consideration of how it affects me personally. That is, however I decide to act, I should not weigh too heavily the ramifications for me professionally. (Hendricks, this volume, p. 97)

The message is straightforward: Sometimes our profession calls upon us to take hard actions that can make our lives uncomfortable. Put more starkly, the ethical evaluator does what the ethical evaluator has to do. We have now entered into the realm of what is often referred to as "moral courage." Acts of moral courage incorporate three components: They reflect a commitment to ethical principles, the actor is aware of the personal danger involved in supporting those principles, and the actor is willing to endure that danger (Kidder, 2005; see also

Austin, Rankel, Kagan, Bergum, & Lemermeyer, 2005). To be sure, there are steps we can take to prepare ourselves for situations in which such courage is required: reading accounts of the courage displayed by others, especially in our own field; developing skills to engage in potentially conflictful interactions; cultivating networks of friends and colleagues who can provide support; and having a well-articulated and strongly held set of personal values are just a few examples. For some evaluators, keeping an ethics journal during projects (Morris, 2004) can help link these values to challenges encountered in a particular evaluation, especially if trusted peers are available for consultation and advice (Gottlieb, 2006). Maintaining a journal can be particularly useful for new evaluators, allowing them to keep track of, and reflect upon, ethical issues that arise during the course of a project. In the end, of course, there is no avoiding the fact that, by definition, moral courage requires the leap of faith—and potential personal sacrifice—associated with doing the right thing simply *because* it is the right thing to do. Reflection must be transformed into action.

Context is also important to consider here. The more one depends on evaluation-related income for his or her livelihood, the greater the personal risk posed by any particular ethical problem encountered in an evaluation, all other things being equal. Thus, a full-time solo practitioner of evaluation is likely to face more "opportunities" to display moral courage than a part-time evaluator whose primary employment is elsewhere. It will be financially easier for the latter evaluator to take the ethical "high road" when responding to challenges, because the loss of that project (e.g., as a result of being fired or terminating the contract) would not represent as big a blow to the individual's base income. It is interesting in this context to note that, in their study of evaluators' perceptions of ethical case scenarios, Morris and Jacobs (2000) found that respondents whose primary employment was in private business/consulting were less likely than those in other settings to find ethical fault with the behavior of the evaluators depicted in the scenarios. The economic realities experienced by those in private business/consulting may produce heightened tolerance and empathy when rendering ethical judgments on the conduct of fellow evaluators. At the same time, Morris (2003) cautions that self-employed evaluators "need to be particularly sensitive to any tendency on their part to generate self-serving rationalizations for their ethical decision-making" (p. 320). One might even argue that when moral courage is called for, the search for such rationalizations is likely to be most intense.

APPLYING THE LESSONS

Ultimately, the goal of analyzing ethics cases in evaluation, at least for practitioners, is to enhance the ethical quality of their professional work. The most detailed strategic framework for ethical decision making in evaluation has been developed by Newman and Brown (1996) and is an especially valuable resource (see also Morris, 2003, 2004). This chapter concludes with a set of guiding questions, mainly based on the themes identified in the chapter, that evaluators can employ when managing the ethical dimensions of their work.

• What can I do during the entry/contracting phase to set the proper ethical tone for this evaluation? To what extent are key stakeholders familiar with the ethical principles that will govern my behavior during the project and influence my expectations of them? To what extent am I familiar with their ethical expectations of me? What ethical "land mines" should I be watchful for in this evaluation, given the distinctive characteristics of the program, setting, and stakeholders involved?

• When I review the Guiding Principles for Evaluators and the Program Evaluation Standards, are there any that stand out as having particular relevance to the evaluation I'm about to embark upon? Are there case studies in the evaluation literature (e.g., from the Ethical Challenges section of the *American Journal of Evaluation*) that describe situations similar to the one I will be encountering? What can I learn from them about how evaluators prioritize principles and standards when facing ethical challenges in these contexts?

• When an ethical problem arises, what steps can I take to ensure that the difficult conversations that need to occur with relevant stakeholders actually take place? How can I maximize the information and perspectives available to inform decision making without losing sight of the fundamental ethical principles that should provide the basis for my actions as an evaluator? Am I able to distinguish between ethical disagreements that reflect disparities in expertise/knowledge versus those that are rooted in value (and perhaps cultural) differences? How can I respond to that distinction in a way that respects the dignity of stakeholders?

• Do I have colleagues to whom I can turn for advice when confronted with an ethical dilemma? How much information about the dilemma is appropriate to share with them? Am I seeking out colleagues whose values and beliefs are so similar to mine that they will simply echo my own views of how I should respond to the problem?

• What does experience teach me about the ethical blind spots that I might bring to this evaluation? What can I do to counteract them as the evaluation unfolds? How can I make stakeholders feel comfortable (or at least less uncomfortable) in sharing with me any concerns they may have about my ethical conduct as an evaluator? What can I do to minimize my defensiveness if such concerns are raised?

• What personal values, ideologies, and cultural assumptions do I carry with me that are likely to be engaged by this evaluation? To what degree do I need to communicate them to stakeholders? How can I communicate what I need to without overwhelming, intimidating, or alienating stakeholders? Am I bringing an ideological "agenda" to this project that is so strong that the conclusions I am likely to reach in the evaluation are preordained? Do I have sufficient knowledge of, and empathy for, the culture of the evaluation setting that I can conduct a competent and fair-minded evaluation? Is my empathy so high that it threatens to bias my evaluation in a positive direction?

• What evidence do I have of how I respond when encountering situations that call for courageous behavior? Do I generally follow the path of least resistance? Do I tend to misinterpret circumstances in a melodramatic fashion that needlessly raises, or appears to raise, the ethical stakes involved? Is this evaluation likely to present challenges that would almost certainly exceed my ability to confront them in an ethical way? Should I agree to conduct such an evaluation?

These questions are not necessarily easy to answer. Indeed, in certain cases it may be impossible to definitively answer many of them. As one gains experience in evaluation, however, the ratio of unanswerable questions to answerable ones is likely to decrease. The value of these questions resides as much in the process of exploring them as it does in the answers that are arrived at. In this respect, they are similar to case scenarios, in which the analysis of the challenge is just as important as the recommendations that emerge, if not more so. Both the process and the product of the activity enhance the ability of evaluators to conduct themselves ethically.

Of course, thinking systematically about ethical issues, whether via case studies or some other device, does not guarantee that evaluation practice will become more ethical. Rather, it contributes to the foundation that supports and informs such practice. This is an essential task if evaluation is to mature as a profession.

REFERENCES

Argyris, C. (1985). *Strategy, change, and defensive routines.* Boston: Pitman.

Austin, W., Rankel, M., Kagan, L., Bergum, V., & Lemermeyer, G. (2005). To stay or to go, to speak or stay silent, to act or not act: Moral distress as experienced by psychologists. *Ethics and Behavior, 15,* 197–212.

Block, P. (2000). *Flawless consulting: A guide to getting your expertise used* (2nd ed.). San Francisco: Jossey-Bass/Pfeiffer.

Datta, L. (2002). The case of the uncertain bridge. *American Journal of Evaluation, 23,* 187–197.

Gottlieb, M. C. (2006). A template for peer ethics consultation. *Ethics and Behavior, 16,* 151–162.

Joint Committee on Standards for Educational Evaluation. (1994). *The program evaluation standards: How to assess evaluations of educational programs* (2nd ed.). Thousand Oaks, CA: Sage.

Kidder, R. M. (2005). *Moral courage.* New York: William Morrow.

Morris, M. (2003). Ethical considerations in evaluation. In T. Kellaghan & D. L. Stufflebeam (Eds.), *International handbook of educational evaluation: Part one. Perspectives* (pp. 303–328). Dordrecht, The Netherlands: Kluwer Academic.

Morris, M. (2004). Not drinking the poison you name: Reflections on teaching ethics to evaluators in for-profit settings. *Evaluation and Program Planning, 27,* 365–369.

Morris, M., & Jacobs, L. (2000). You got a problem with that? Exploring evaluators' disagreements about ethics. *Evaluation Review, 24,* 384–406.

Newman, D. L, & Brown, R. D. (1996). *Applied ethics for program evaluation.* Thousand Oaks, CA: Sage.

Paasche-Orlow, M. (2004). The ethics of cultural competence. *Academic Medicine, 29,* 347–350.

Strike, K. A., Anderson, M. S., Curren, R., van Geel, T., Pritchard, I., & Robertson, E. (2002). *Ethical standards of the American Educational Research Association: Cases and commentary.* Washington, DC: American Educational Research Association.

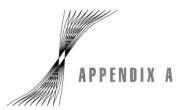

APPENDIX A

The Guiding Principles for Evaluators

A. Systematic Inquiry: Evaluators conduct systematic, data-based inquiries.

1. To ensure the accuracy and credibility of the evaluative information they produce, evaluators should adhere to the highest technical standards appropriate to the methods they use.

2. Evaluators should explore with the client the shortcomings and strengths both of the various evaluation questions and the various approaches that might be used for answering those questions.

3. Evaluators should communicate their methods and approaches accurately and in sufficient detail to allow others to understand, interpret and critique their work. They should make clear the limitations of an evaluation and its results. Evaluators should discuss in a contextually appropriate way those values, assumptions, theories, methods, results, and analyses significantly affecting the interpretation of the evaluative findings. These statements apply to all aspects of the evaluation, from its initial conceptualization to the eventual use of findings.

B. Competence: Evaluators provide competent performance to stakeholders.

1. Evaluators should possess (or ensure that the evaluation team possesses) the education, abilities, skills and experience appropriate to undertake the tasks proposed in the evaluation.

2. To ensure recognition, accurate interpretation and respect for diversity, evaluators should ensure that the members of the evaluation team collectively demonstrate cultural competence. Cultural competence

Source: American Evaluation Association (*www.eval.org/Publications/GuidingPrinciples. asp*).

would be reflected in evaluators seeking awareness of their own culturally-based assumptions, their understanding of the worldviews of culturally-different participants and stakeholders in the evaluation, and the use of appropriate evaluation strategies and skills in working with culturally different groups. Diversity may be in terms of race, ethnicity, gender, religion, socio-economics, or other factors pertinent to the evaluation context.

3. Evaluators should practice within the limits of their professional training and competence, and should decline to conduct evaluations that fall substantially outside those limits. When declining the commission or request is not feasible or appropriate, evaluators should make clear any significant limitations on the evaluation that might result. Evaluators should make every effort to gain the competence directly or through the assistance of others who possess the required expertise.

4. Evaluators should continually seek to maintain and improve their competencies, in order to provide the highest level of performance in their evaluations. This continuing professional development might include formal coursework and workshops, self-study, evaluations of one's own practice, and working with other evaluators to learn from their skills and expertise.

C. **Integrity/Honesty:** Evaluators display honesty and integrity in their own behavior, and attempt to ensure the honesty and integrity of the entire evaluation process.

1. Evaluators should negotiate honestly with clients and relevant stakeholders concerning the costs, tasks to be undertaken, limitations of methodology, scope of results likely to be obtained, and uses of data resulting from a specific evaluation. It is primarily the evaluator's responsibility to initiate discussion and clarification of these matters, not the client's.

2. Before accepting an evaluation assignment, evaluators should disclose any roles or relationships they have that might pose a conflict of interest (or appearance of a conflict) with their role as an evaluator. If they proceed with the evaluation, the conflict(s) should be clearly articulated in reports of the evaluation results.

3. Evaluators should record all changes made in the originally negotiated project plans, and the reasons why the changes were made. If those changes would significantly affect the scope and likely results of the evaluation, the evaluator should inform the client and other important stakeholders in a timely fashion (barring good reason to the contrary, before proceeding with further work) of the changes and their likely impact.

4. Evaluators should be explicit about their own, their clients', and other stakeholders' interests and values concerning the conduct and outcomes of an evaluation.

5. Evaluators should not misrepresent their procedures, data or findings. Within reasonable limits, they should attempt to prevent or correct misuse of their work by others.

6. If evaluators determine that certain procedures or activities are likely to produce misleading evaluative information or conclusions, they have the responsibility to communicate their concerns and the reasons for them. If discussions with the client do not resolve these concerns, the evaluator should decline to conduct the evaluation. If declining the assignment is unfeasible or inappropriate, the evaluator should consult colleagues or relevant stakeholders about other proper ways to proceed. (Options might include discussions at a higher level, a dissenting cover letter or appendix, or refusal to sign the final document.)

7. Evaluators should disclose all sources of financial support for an evaluation, and the source of the request for the evaluation.

D. **Respect for People:** Evaluators respect the security, dignity and self-worth of respondents, program participants, clients, and other evaluation stakeholders.

1. Evaluators should seek a comprehensive understanding of the important contextual elements of the evaluation. Contextual factors that may influence the results of a study include geographic location, timing, political and social climate, economic conditions, and other relevant activities in progress at the same time.

2. Evaluators should abide by current professional ethics, standards, and regulations regarding risks, harms, and burdens that might befall those participating in the evaluation; regarding informed consent for participation in evaluation; and regarding informing participants and clients about the scope and limits of confidentiality.

3. Because justified negative or critical conclusions from an evaluation must be explicitly stated, evaluations sometimes produce results that harm client or stakeholder interests. Under this circumstance, evaluators should seek to maximize the benefits and reduce any unnecessary harms that might occur, provided this will not compromise the integrity of the evaluation findings. Evaluators should carefully judge when the benefits from doing the evaluation or in performing certain evaluation procedures should be forgone because of the risks or harms. To the extent possible, these issues should be anticipated during the negotiation of the evaluation.

4. Knowing that evaluations may negatively affect the interests of some stakeholders, evaluators should conduct the evaluation and communicate its results in a way that clearly respects the stakeholders' dignity and self-worth.

5. Where feasible, evaluators should attempt to foster social equity in evaluation, so that those who give to the evaluation may benefit in

return. For example, evaluators should seek to ensure that those who bear the burdens of contributing data and incurring any risks do so willingly, and that they have full knowledge of and opportunity to obtain any benefits of the evaluation. Program participants should be informed that their eligibility to receive services does not hinge on their participation in the evaluation.

6. Evaluators have the responsibility to understand and respect differences among participants, such as differences in their culture, religion, gender, disability, age, sexual orientation and ethnicity, and to account for potential implications of these differences when planning, conducting, analyzing, and reporting evaluations.

E. **Responsibilities for General and Public Welfare:** Evaluators articulate and take into account the diversity of general and public interests and values that may be related to the evaluation.

1. When planning and reporting evaluations, evaluators should include relevant perspectives and interests of the full range of stakeholders.

2. Evaluators should consider not only the immediate operations and outcomes of whatever is being evaluated, but also its broad assumptions, implications and potential side effects.

3. Freedom of information is essential in a democracy. Evaluators should allow all relevant stakeholders access to evaluative information in forms that respect people and honor promises of confidentiality. Evaluators should actively disseminate information to stakeholders as resources allow. Communications that are tailored to a given stakeholder should include all results that may bear on interests of that stakeholder and refer to any other tailored communications to other stakeholders. In all cases, evaluators should strive to present results clearly and simply so that clients and other stakeholders can easily understand the evaluation process and results.

4. Evaluators should maintain a balance between client needs and other needs. Evaluators necessarily have a special relationship with the client who funds or requests the evaluation. By virtue of that relationship, evaluators must strive to meet legitimate client needs whenever it is feasible and appropriate to do so. However, that relationship can also place evaluators in difficult dilemmas when client interests conflict with other interests, or when client interests conflict with the obligation of evaluators for systematic inquiry, competence, integrity, and respect for people. In these cases, evaluators should explicitly identify and discuss the conflicts with the client and relevant stakeholders, resolve them when possible, determine whether continued work on the evaluation is advisable if the conflicts cannot be resolved, and make clear any significant limitations on the evaluation that might result if the conflict is not resolved.

5. Evaluators have obligations that encompass the public interest and good. These obligations are especially important when evaluators are supported by publicly-generated funds; but clear threats to the public good should never be ignored in any evaluation. Because the public interest and good are rarely the same as the interests of any particular group (including those of the client or funder), evaluators will usually have to go beyond analysis of particular stakeholder interests and consider the welfare of society as a whole.

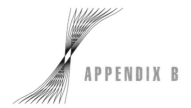

The Program Evaluation Standards, Second Edition

SUMMARY OF THE STANDARDS

Utility Standards

The utility standards are intended to ensure that an evaluation will serve the information needs of intended users.

U1 Stakeholder Identification Persons involved in or affected by the evaluation should be identified, so that their needs can be addressed.

U2 Evaluator Credibility The persons conducting the evaluation should be both trustworthy and competent to perform the evaluation, so that the evaluation findings achieve maximum credibility and acceptance.

U3 Information Scope and Selection Information collected should be broadly selected to address pertinent questions about the program and be responsive to the needs and interests of clients and other specified stakeholders.

U4 Values Identification The perspectives, procedures, and rationale used to interpret the findings should be carefully described, so that the bases for value judgments are clear.

U5 Report Clarity Evaluation reports should clearly describe the program being evaluated, including its context, and the purposes, procedures, and find-

Source: Joint Committee on Standards for Educational Evaluation (*www.wmich.edu/evalctr/ jc/PGMSTNDS-SUM.htm*).

ings of the evaluation, so that essential information is provided and easily understood.

U6 Report Timeliness and Dissemination Significant interim findings and evaluation reports should be disseminated to intended users, so that they can be used in a timely fashion.

U7 Evaluation Impact Evaluations should be planned, conducted, and reported in ways that encourage follow-through by stakeholders, so that the likelihood that the evaluation will be used is increased.

Feasibility Standards

The feasibility standards are intended to ensure that an evaluation will be realistic, prudent, diplomatic, and frugal.

F1 Practical Procedures The evaluation procedures should be practical, to keep disruption to a minimum while needed information is obtained.

F2 Political Viability The evaluation should be planned and conducted with anticipation of the different positions of various interest groups, so that their cooperation may be obtained, and so that possible attempts by any of these groups to curtail evaluation operations or to bias or misapply the results can be averted or counteracted.

F3 Cost Effectiveness The evaluation should be efficient and produce information of sufficient value, so that the resources expended can be justified.

Propriety Standards

The propriety standards are intended to ensure that an evaluation will be conducted legally, ethically, and with due regard for the welfare of those involved in the evaluation, as well as those affected by its results.

P1 Service Orientation Evaluations should be designed to assist organizations to address and effectively serve the needs of the full range of targeted participants.

P2 Formal Agreements Obligations of the formal parties to an evaluation (what is to be done, how, by whom, when) should be agreed to in writing, so that these parties are obligated to adhere to all conditions of the agreement or formally to renegotiate it.

P3 Rights of Human Subjects Evaluations should be designed and conducted to respect and protect the rights and welfare of human subjects.

P4 Human Interactions Evaluators should respect human dignity and worth in their interactions with other persons associated with an evaluation, so that participants are not threatened or harmed.

P5 Complete and Fair Assessment The evaluation should be complete and fair in its examination and recording of strengths and weaknesses of the program being evaluated, so that strengths can be built upon and problem areas addressed.

P6 Disclosure of Findings The formal parties to an evaluation should ensure that the full set of evaluation findings along with pertinent limitations are made accessible to the persons affected by the evaluation and any others with expressed legal rights to receive the results.

P7 Conflict of Interest Conflict of interest should be dealt with openly and honestly, so that it does not compromise the evaluation processes and results.

P8 Fiscal Responsibility The evaluator's allocation and expenditure of resources should reflect sound accountability procedures and otherwise be prudent and ethically responsible, so that expenditures are accounted for and appropriate.

Accuracy Standards

The accuracy standards are intended to ensure that an evaluation will reveal and convey technically adequate information about the features that determine worth or merit of the program being evaluated.

A1 Program Documentation The program being evaluated should be described and documented clearly and accurately, so that the program is clearly identified.

A2 Context Analysis The context in which the program exists should be examined in enough detail, so that its likely influences on the program can be identified.

A3 Described Purposes and Procedures The purposes and procedures of the evaluation should be monitored and described in enough detail, so that they can be identified and assessed.

A4 Defensible Information Sources The sources of information used in a program evaluation should be described in enough detail, so that the adequacy of the information can be assessed.

A5 Valid Information The information-gathering procedures should be chosen or developed and then implemented so that they will assure that the interpretation arrived at is valid for the intended use.

A6 Reliable Information The information-gathering procedures should be chosen or developed and then implemented so that they will assure that the information obtained is sufficiently reliable for the intended use.

A7 Systematic Information The information collected, processed, and reported in an evaluation should be systematically reviewed, and any errors found should be corrected.

A8 Analysis of Quantitative Information Quantitative information in an evaluation should be appropriately and systematically analyzed so that evaluation questions are effectively answered.

A9 Analysis of Qualitative Information Qualitative information in an evaluation should be appropriately and systematically analyzed so that evaluation questions are effectively answered.

A10 Justified Conclusions The conclusions reached in an evaluation should be explicitly justified, so that stakeholders can assess them.

A11 Impartial Reporting Reporting procedures should guard against distortion caused by personal feelings and biases of any party to the evaluation, so that evaluation reports fairly reflect the evaluation findings.

A12 Metaevaluation The evaluation itself should be formatively and summatively evaluated against these and other pertinent standards, so that its conduct is appropriately guided and, on completion, stakeholders can closely examine its strengths and weaknesses.

Author Index

Subject Index

"f" following a page number indicates a figure;
"t" following a page number indicates a table.

219

About the Editor

Michael Morris is Professor of Psychology at the University of New Haven, where he directs the Master's Program in Community Psychology. He served as the first editor of the Ethical Challenges section of the *American Journal of Evaluation* from 1998 to 2004. His publications have appeared in *Evaluation Review, Evaluation and Program Planning,* the *American Journal of Community Psychology,* and the *Journal of Community of Psychology,* among others. He coedited, with Jody Fitzpatrick, the *New Directions for Evaluation* volume devoted to "Current and Emerging Ethical Challenges in Evaluation" (1999). Dr. Morris is a member of the Editorial Advisory Boards of *New Directions for Evaluation* and the *American Journal of Evaluation* and has served as Chair of the Ethics Committee and the Public Affairs Committee of the American Evaluation Association. His other books include *Poverty and Public Policy* (with John Williamson) and *Myths about the Powerless* (with M. Brinton Lykes, Ramsay Liem, and Ali Banuazizi). A trainer in evaluation ethics throughout the United States and abroad, he received his PhD in community–social psychology from Boston College.

Contributors

Gail V. Barrington has a doctorate in educational administration from the University of Alberta. A certified management consultant, she established the Barrington Research Group, Inc., in 1985. Dr. Barrington has conducted over 100 program evaluations, primarily in health and education. In 2006 she coedited the issue of *New Directions for Evaluation* devoted to "Independent Evaluation Consulting." She has published articles in evaluation journals and is the author of several entries in the *Encyclopedia of Evaluation* (Sage, 2005). In 1992 she received the Division H Annual Evaluation Report Award from the American Educational Research Association for her report on integrated services in education. She is a member of the American Evaluation Association's Board of Directors, former chair of the AEA Ethics Committee, and a founding director of the Canadian Evaluation Society Education Fund.

David M. Chavis, whose PhD is in community psychology from Vanderbilt University, is president of the Association for the Study and Development of Community. He is internationally recognized for his work on the implementation, support, and evaluation of community initiatives. He has received a Distinguished Career Award from the American Psychological Association and the award for Outstanding Evaluation of the Year from the American Evaluation Association. The primary focus of his practice has been the relationship between community development and the prevention of poverty, violence, substance abuse, illness, and other social problems through community capacity building. He has led evaluations of collaborative community initiatives for the White House Office for National Drug Control Policy, the U.S. Department of Justice, the U.S. Center for Substance Abuse Prevention, the Annie E. Casey Foundation, the Robert Wood Johnson Foundation, and other national and local organizations. Dr. Chavis is also a consultant, writer, and trainer on the evaluation of collaborative efforts.

Leslie J. Cooksy obtained her PhD in human service studies at Cornell University, majoring in program evaluation and public policy, and has been a professional evaluator for 15 years. She is an Associate Professor at the University of Delaware, where she coordinates an interdisciplinary graduate evaluation program in the College of Human Services, Education, and Public Policy. Her previous positions include director of the Tobacco Control Evaluation Center at the University of California, Davis; senior social science analyst in the Program Evaluation and Methodology Division of the U.S. Government Accountability Office; and director of the Center for Community Research and Service at the University of Delaware. Her areas of expertise include evaluation quality and metaevaluation, as well as the use of logic models in evaluation. Dr. Cooksy serves as the editor of the Ethical Challenges section of the *American Journal of Evaluation* and is on the Editorial Advisory Board of *New Directions for Evaluation*. Her work has been published in *Public Administration Review*, the *American Journal of Evaluation*, and *Evaluation and Program Planning*, among others. She is a past recipient of the American Evaluation Association's Marcia Guttentag Award for early career contributions to evaluation practice.

sarita davis earned her PhD in program evaluation from Cornell University and is currently an Associate Professor in the Whitney M. Young, Jr. School of Social Work at Clark Atlanta University. A recipient of the University's Claudette Rivers-King Excellence Award in both 1999 and 2005, Dr. davis's primary areas of scholarship are HIV/AIDS in the Black community, African-centered research methods, and community-based evaluation. She recently cofounded African Women in Research and Evaluation, a grassroots organization focusing on the integration of evaluation, practice, and research in urban settings.

Michael Hendricks is an independent evaluation consultant currently based in Bethesda, Maryland. After receiving his PhD from Northwestern University in methodology and evaluation research, he served as an evaluation official for the U.S. Department of Health and Human Services. As a consultant for the past 22 years, he has worked with a wide variety of clients, including governments at all levels (city, county, state, and national), international development agencies in numerous countries, national nonprofit associations, foundations, and local service delivery agencies. The primary thrust of his professional practice is to help human service programs function as effectively and efficiently as possible. Dr. Hendricks is also a trainer in areas such as research analysis, both in the United States and abroad, and serves on the Editorial Advisory Board of the *American Journal of Evaluation.*

Karen E. Kirkhart holds a PhD in social work and psychology from the University of Michigan and is currently Professor in the School of Social Work, College of Human Services and Health Professions, at Syracuse University. She has taught, practiced, and written about evaluation for nearly three decades, with an emphasis on evaluation theory. Dr. Kirkhart's work on multicultural validity examines the many ways in which culture bounds understanding in general and judgments of program merit and worth in particular. Her work on evaluation influence places evaluation use within the broader context of power, influence, and consequences, interweaving ethics and validity. Dr. Kirkhart, a former president of the American Evaluation Association, received the 2006 Recognition Award from the Multiethnic Issues Topical Interest Group of the AEA. Her chapter "Through a Cultural Lens: Reflections on Validity and Theory in Evaluation" appears in *The Role of Culture and Cultural Context: A Mandate for Inclusion, the Discovery of Truth, and Understanding in Evaluative Theory and Practice,* edited by Stafford Hood, Rodney Hopson, and Henry Frierson (Information Age, 2005).

Laura C. Leviton has been a senior program officer of the Robert Wood Johnson Foundation in Princeton, New Jersey, since 1999, overseeing 44 evaluations and $68 million in research to date. She was formerly a professor at two schools of public health, where she collaborated on the first randomized experiment on HIV prevention and later on two large, place-based randomized experiments on improving medical practices. She received the 1993 award from the American Psychological Association for Distinguished Contributions to Psychology in the Public Interest. She has served on two Institute of Medicine committees and the National Advisory Committee on HIV and STD Prevention. Dr. Leviton was president of the American Evaluation Association in 2000 and has coauthored two books: *Foundations of Program Evaluation* and *Confronting Public Health Risks.* She is interested in all aspects of evaluation practice. She received her PhD in social psychology from the University of Kansas.

Melvin M. Mark, who received his PhD in social psychology from Northwestern University, is Professor of Psychology at the Pennsylvania State University. He has served as editor of the *American Journal of Evaluation* and is now editor emeritus. Dr. Mark was president of the American Evaluation Association in 2006. His interests include the theory, methodology, practice, and profession of program and policy evaluation. His evaluation experience encompasses prevention programs, federal personnel policies, and educational interventions, among other areas. Dr. Mark's books include *Evaluation: An Integrated Frame-*

work for Understanding, Guiding, and Improving Policies and Programs (Jossey-Bass, 2000; with Gary Henry and George Julnes) and *The SAGE Handbook of Evaluation* (Sage, 2006; with Ian Shaw and Jennifer Greene). His current work includes the forthcoming volumes *Exemplars of Evaluation* (Sage; with Jody Fitzpatrick and Tina Christie) and *Social Psychology and Evaluation* (Guilford Press; with Stewart Donaldson and Bernadette Campbell).

Michael Morris (see "About the Editor").

Lucía Orellana-Damacela received her master's degree from Loyola University, Chicago, and is currently working on her doctoral dissertation. Her background as an applied social psychologist has been used primarily in the areas of planning and evaluation with social service organizations. She emphasizes the fostering of evaluation understanding and capacity, the promotion of utilization of evaluation results, and the use of participation to increase evaluation's relevance, accuracy, and stakeholder ownership. Her publications include "Implementing an Outcomes Model in the Participatory Evaluation of Community Initiatives" (*Journal of Prevention and Intervention in the Community*, 2003) and "Experiences of Differential Treatment among College Students of Color" (*Journal of Higher Education*, 2003).

Sharon F. Rallis is Dwight W. Allen Distinguished Professor of Education Policy and Reform at the University of Massachusetts at Amherst, where she is also director of the Center for Education Policy and teaches courses on inquiry, program evaluation, qualitative methodology, and organizational theory. Her doctorate is from Harvard University. A past president of the American Evaluation Association, Dr. Rallis studies and writes about policy, leadership, and inquiry and has been evaluating education programs for nearly three decades. Her current research focuses on the local implementation of programs driven by federal, state, or district policies, and she recently collaborated on a book explicating moral reasoning behind policy decisions of school principals (*Leading Dynamic Schools: How to Create and Implement Ethical Policies*, Corwin Press). Dr. Rallis is coauthor, with Gretchen Rossman, of *Learning in the Field: An Introduction to Qualitative Research* (Sage) and has published in *New Directions for Evaluation* as well as in other books on evaluation.

Mary Ann Scheirer, who holds a PhD in sociology from Cornell University, is currently an independent consultant with her own firm, Scheirer Consulting. She retired in 2003 from the Robert Wood Johnson Foundation, where she was a senior program officer for research and evaluation. Previously, she was an independent consultant for the evaluation of health promotion, substance abuse, education, and human services programs. She has published extensively on process evaluation, including assessing program implementation and sustainability, and has assisted many agencies with the development of performance measures. Dr. Scheirer has served on the Boards of Directors of the American Evaluation Association and the Consumer Health Foundation and has been president of Washington Evaluators.

William R. Shadish is Professor and founding faculty at the University of California, Merced. He received his PhD in clinical psychology from Purdue University and completed a postdoctoral fellowship in methodology and program evaluation at Northwestern University. His research interests include experimental and quasi-experimental design, the empirical study of methodological issues, the methodology and practice of meta-analysis, and evaluation theory. He is coauthor of *Experimental and Quasi-Experimental Designs for Generalized Causal Inference* (with Thomas D. Cook and Donald T. Campbell, 2002), *Foundations of Program Evaluation* (with Thomas D. Cook and Laura C. Leviton, 1991), and *ES: A Computer Program and Manual for Effect Size Calculation* (with Leslie Robinson and Congxiao Lu, 1997); coeditor of five other volumes; and the author of over 100 articles and chapters. He was president of the American Evaluation Association in 1997 and winner of AEA's Paul F. Lazarsfeld Award for Evaluation Theory in 1994, the Robert Ingle Award for service to AEA in 2000, the Outstanding Research Publication Award from the American Association for Marriage and Family Therapy in 1994 and 1996, and the Donald T. Campbell Award for Innovations in Methodology from the Policy Studies Organization in 2002. Dr. Shadish is associate editor of *Multivariate Behavioral Research* and a past editor of *New Directions for Evaluation*.

Yolanda Suarez-Balcazar received her PhD in developmental and community psychology from the University of Kansas. She is Professor and head of the Department of Occupational Therapy at the University of Illinois at Chicago, where she also serves as associate director of the Center for Capacity Building on Minorities with Disabilities Research. Her research expertise includes the study of participatory and empowerment evaluation of community initiatives, university–community partnerships, participatory needs assessment methodologies with people with disabilities, and issues of multicultural training and diversity. Her publications in these areas include the volumes *Empowerment and Participatory Evaluation of Community Interventions: Multiple Benefits* (coedited with Gary W. Harper, 2003) and *Participatory Community Research: Theory and Methods in Action* (coauthored with Leonard A. Jason, Christopher B. Keys, Renee Taylor, and Margaret Davis, 2003). She is a fellow of the American Psychological Association and recipient of the 2005 Minority Mentorship Award from the Society for Community Research and Action.